The British Medical Association

FAMILY DOCTOR

THYROID DISORDERS

The British Medical Association

FAMILY DOCTOR GUIDE *to*

THYROID DISORDERS

DR. ANTHONY TOFT

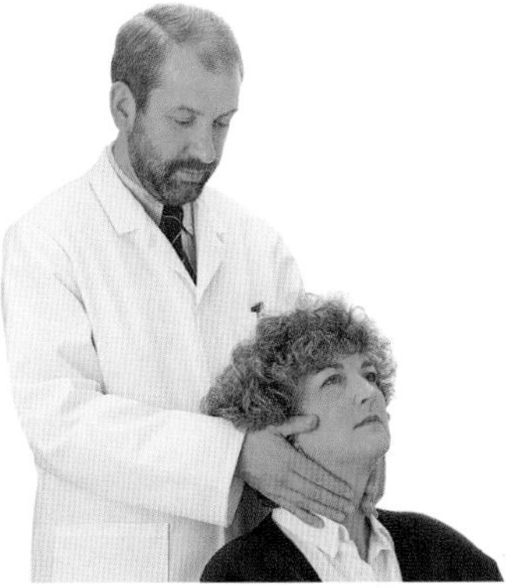

MEDICAL EDITOR
DR. TONY SMITH

DORLING KINDERSLEY
LONDON • NEW YORK • SYDNEY • MOSCOW
www.dk.com

IMPORTANT

This book is not designed as a substitute for personal medical advice but as a supplement to that advice for the patient who wishes to understand more about his/her condition.

Before taking any form of treatment **YOU SHOULD ALWAYS CONSULT YOUR MEDICAL PRACTITIONER.**

In particular (without limit) you should note that advances in medical science occur rapidly and some of the information contained in this book about drugs and treatment may very soon be out of date.

PLEASE NOTE
The author regrets that he cannot enter into any correspondence with readers.

A DORLING KINDERSLEY BOOK
www.dk.com

Senior Editor Mary Lindsay
Senior Designer Sarah Hall
Production Assistant Elizabeth Cherry

Managing Editor Stephanie Jackson
Managing Art Editor Nigel Duffield

Produced for Dorling Kindersley Limited by
Design Revolution, Queens Park Villa,
30 West Drive, Brighton, East Sussex BN2 2GE
Editorial Director Ian Whitelaw
Art Director Fiona Roberts
Editor Julie Whitaker
Designer Vanessa Good

Published in Great Britain in 1999 by
Dorling Kindersley Limited,
9 Henrietta Street, London WC2E 8PS

2 4 6 8 10 9 7 5 3 1

A CIP catalogue record for this book is available from the British Library

ISBN 07513 0673 8

Reproduced by Colourscan, Singapore
Printed in Hong Kong by Wing King Tong

Contents

Introduction

The thyroid gland lies in the front of the neck between the skin and the voice box. It has a right and left lobe each about five centimetres in length and joined in the midline. The entire thyroid gland weighs less than 20 grams (about an ounce).

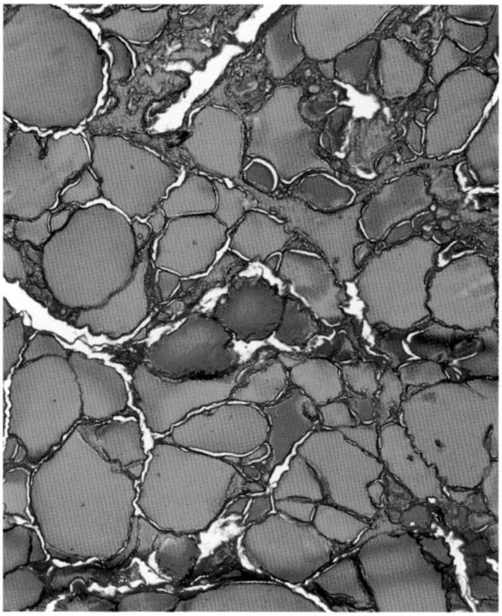

INSIDE THE THYROID
This microscope picture of the thyroid gland shows the thyroid follicles (seen here as blue), collections of cells that produce thyroid hormones. The orange patches are areas of stored hormones.

Despite its small size, the thyroid gland is an extremely important organ that works to control our metabolism and is responsible for the normal working of every cell in the body. It achieves this by manufacturing the hormones known as thyroxine (T4) and triiodothyronine (T3) and secreting these hormones into the bloodstream.

Iodine is an important constituent of these hormones. There are four atoms of iodine in each molecule of thyroxine, hence the abbreviation T4, and three atoms of iodine in each molecule of triiodothyronine or T3. Doctors believe that T4 only starts to be active when it is converted, mainly in the liver, to T3 by the removal of one atom of iodine.

In parts of the world where there is a severe lack of iodine in the diet, such as the Himalayas, there is not enough iodine for the thyroid gland to make adequate amounts of T3 and T4. In an attempt to compensate, the

Location of the Thyroid Gland

This diagram shows the position of the thyroid within the neck. It is a butterfly-shaped gland consisting of two lobes in the lower neck, one on each side of the trachea (windpipe), joined by a connecting layer of thyroid tissue.

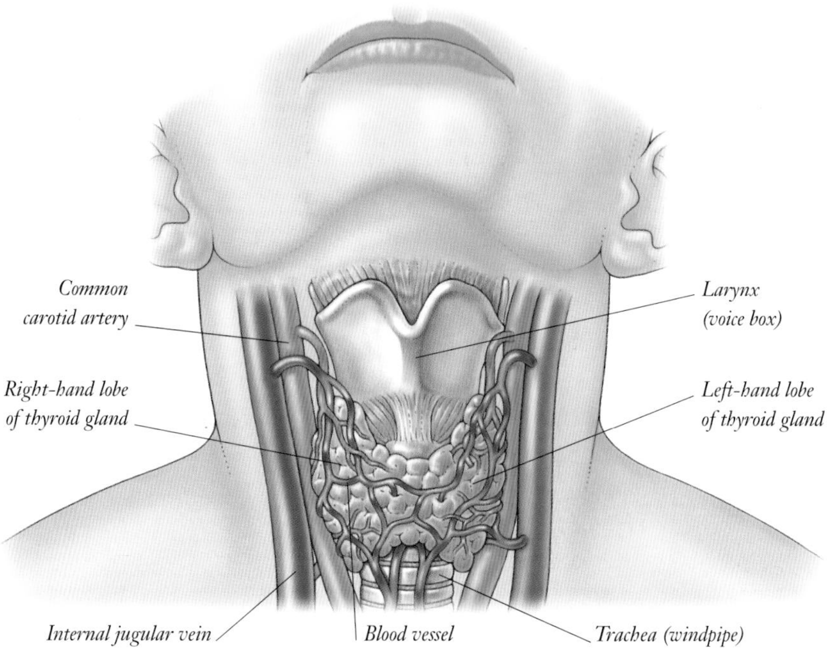

thyroid gland enlarges to form what is known as a goitre, which is visible. If this extra manufacturing capacity is still inadequate, the patient develops an underactive thyroid gland (see p.30). Iodine deficiency is not present in the UK. Sometimes too much iodine in the diet causes the thyroid gland to produce excessive amounts of thyroid hormones. This can also be a result of medication.

In healthy people, the amounts of T3 and T4 in the blood are maintained within narrow limits by a hormone known as thyroid-stimulating hormone (TSH) or thyrotrophin. TSH is secreted by the anterior pituitary gland, which is a pea-sized structure that hangs from the undersurface of the brain just behind the eyes and is enclosed in a bony depression in the base of the skull.

When thyroid disease causes the thyroid hormone levels in the blood to fall, TSH secretion from the pituitary is increased; when thyroid hormone levels rise, TSH secretion is switched off – a relationship known as 'negative feedback', a concept familiar to engineers and biologists.

If your GP suspects that you may have an underactive thyroid gland (hypothyroidism), his or her diagnosis can be confirmed by sending a sample of your blood to the laboratory for analysis. If tests reveal low levels of the hormones T3 and T4 and high levels of TSH in your blood, then your doctor was correct. Similarly, the

Maintaining Normal Hormone Levels

The production of thryoid hormones by the thyroid gland is regulated by the pituitary gland, which produces TSH in response to the levels of thyroid hormones in the bloodstream. This mechanism is known as a 'negative feedback' loop.

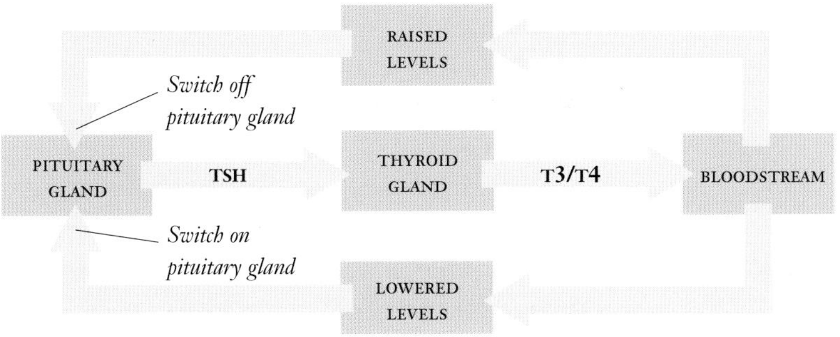

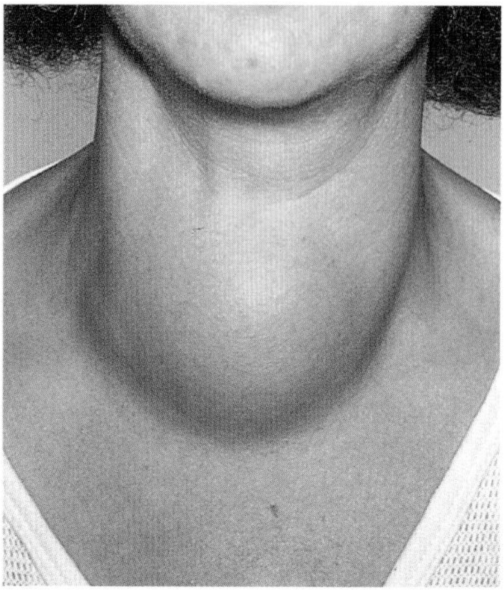

ENLARGED THYROID
Enlargement of the thyroid gland, or goitre, can be caused by iodine deficiency, but this is not a common cause in developed countries.

diagnosis of an overactive thyroid gland (hyperthyroidism) would be confirmed by high levels of T3 and T4 and low levels of TSH. The results of the tests are available within a few days.

Patients who suffer from uncomplicated hypothyroidism will not usually be referred to hospital, and your GP can prescribe and monitor your treatment. Most patients with hyperthyroidism or with abnormal growth of the thyroid gland will be referred to a hospital specialist for further investigation and advice about treatment.

Thyroid disorders are very common, and hyperthyroidism, hypothyroidism or abnormal growth or enlargement of the gland (goitre or thyroid nodule) affects about one in 20 people. Most diseases of the thyroid can be treated successfully, and even thyroid cancer, which is rare, may not lead to a reduction in life expectancy if detected early and treated appropriately.

Thyroid disease often runs in families, but in an unpredictable manner, and certain forms are associated with an increased risk of developing conditions such as diabetes mellitus or pernicious anaemia. All types of thyroid disease are more common in women.

The following chapters will deal with each of the most common thyroid disorders individually.

Case History: **IODINE DEFICIENCY**

Ahmed was born in a village in the high mountains of northern Pakistan where he spent most of his childhood. At the age of 20 he came to London to study engineering. At a routine medical examination, he was noticed to have

Incidence of Iodine-Deficiency Goitre

This world map shows the regions in which iodine-deficiency goitre is a common disorder. The distribution shows primarily those areas where the soil lacks iodine and the diet of the people relies entirely on locally produced food.

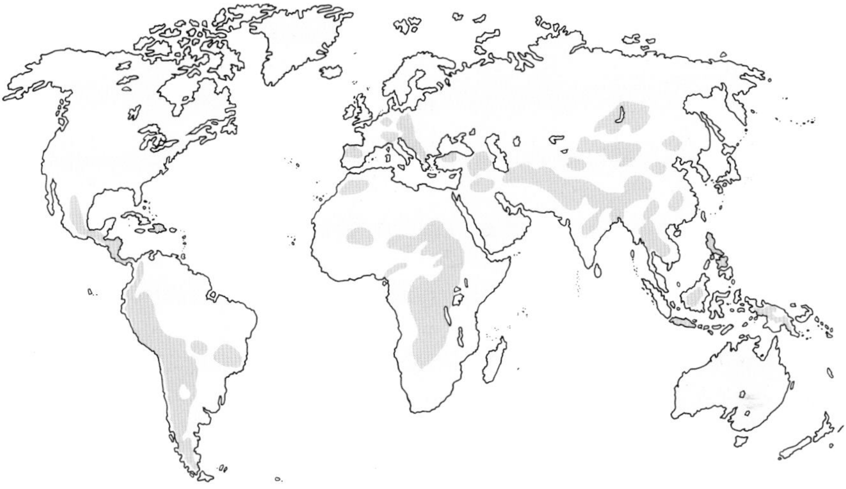

Areas in the world affected by iodine-deficiency goitre

a goitre. He felt well and all the thyroid tests were normal. When Ahmed told the doctor that most of the people in the village where he was born also had a goitre, the cause of the goitre was attributed to iodine deficiency during childhood. His current diet contains enough iodine to prevent the development of hypothyroidism, but his goitre is likely to remain, even though he has decided to live the rest of his life in a part of the world where there is an adequate amount of iodine in the diet.

KEY POINTS

- Thyroid disease is common, affecting around one in 20 people.
- More women than men are affected.
- Your GP can diagnose the condition with a simple blood test.
- Treatment is usually successful, and even thyroid cancer can be cured if caught early.

Overactive thyroid

An overactive thyroid (hyperthyroidism or thyrotoxicosis) results from the overproduction of the thyroid hormones, T4 and T3, by the thyroid gland. In three-quarters of patients this is the result of the presence in the blood of an antibody that stimulates the thyroid, not only to secrete excessive amounts of thyroid hormones but also, in some, to increase the size of the thyroid gland, producing a goitre.

HYPERTHYROIDISM
Anxiety and palpitations are often early symptoms of an overactive thyroid, as well as a feeling of fullness in the neck.

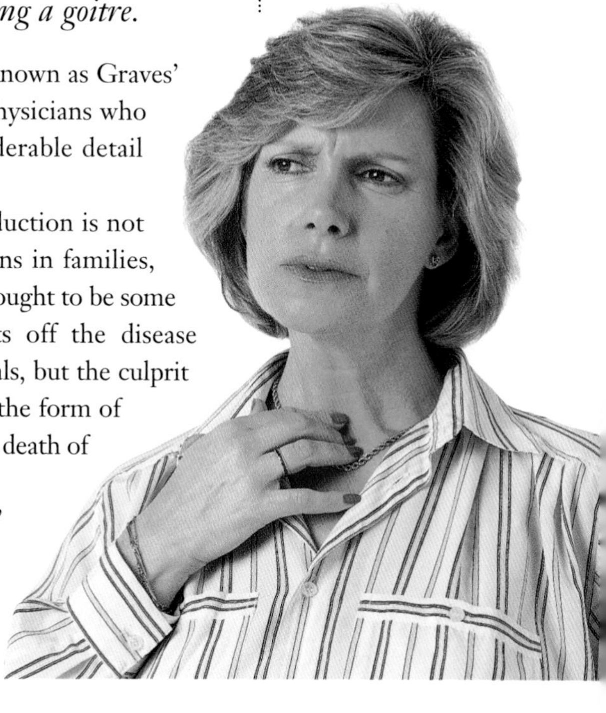

This type of hyperthyroidism is known as Graves' disease, named after one of the physicians who described the condition in considerable detail more than 200 years ago.

The cause of the antibody production is not known but, as Graves' disease runs in families, genes must play a part. There is thought to be some environmental trigger that starts off the disease in genetically susceptible individuals, but the culprit has not been identified. Stress, in the form of major life events such as divorce or death of a close relative, may play a role.

Some patients with Graves' disease develop prominent eyes (proptosis or exophthalmos) and a few also suffer from raised, red, itchy areas of skin on the front of the lower legs or on the top of the feet, which are known as pretibial myxoedema. These, like the production of the thyroid-stimulating antibodies, are caused by an abnormality in the patient's immune system, which doctors do not yet fully understand. Most other patients with hyperthyroidism have a goitre containing one or more nodules or 'lumps'. These over-produce thyroid hormones in their own right and are not under the control of TSH, as is the normal thyroid gland.

Graves' disease can come on at any age but most commonly affects women in the 40- to 50-year-old age group. Between a third and a half of all patients will have a single episode of hyperthyroidism lasting several months. The rest will have successive episodes of hyperthyroidism that will occur over many years. Unfortunately, it is not possible to predict the pattern of hyperthyroidism when it first occurs. Hyperthyroidism resulting from a nodular goitre is unusual before the age of 40 and, unlike some patients with Graves' disease, it persists indefinitely once it has developed.

Symptoms of an Overactive Thyroid

- Weight loss
- Heat intolerance
- Irritability
- Palpitations
- Breathlessness
- Tremor
- Muscle weakness
- Increase in bowel movements
- Irregular menstruation
- Itchy skin, thinning of the hair, brittle nails
- Watering eyes
- Goitre

HOW DOES IT DEVELOP?

In retrospect, most patients will have had symptoms for at least six months before they go to see their doctor, but in some, usually teenagers, the onset is more rapid, with symptoms present for only a few weeks. Not all patients with hyperthyroidism have all the symptoms listed in the box above. In elderly people, the predominant features, in addition to weight loss, are often a reduction in appetite, muscle weakness and apathy. A young woman, on the other hand, may appear to be full of energy and be unable to sit still for more than a few seconds.

WHAT ARE THE SYMPTOMS?

An overactive thyroid gland causes the chemical reactions in the body to speed up, producing mental as well as physical symptoms.

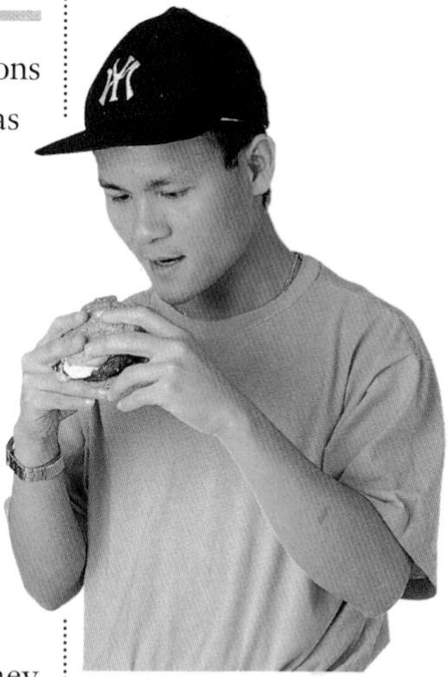

INCREASED APPETITE
People with an overactive thyroid may find that despite eating much more than usual, they still lose weight.

WEIGHT LOSS

This happens to almost all patients as a result of a 'burning off' of calories caused by the high levels of thyroid hormones in the blood. You will probably find you're hungry all the time, and that you even have to get up in the night to get something to eat. The weight loss can range from 2–3 kilograms up to as much as 35 kilograms or more, but a few people find that their appetite increases to such an extent that they may gain a little weight. If you are severely overweight when the condition first starts, you'll probably be delighted to find that you're losing weight and put it down to dieting, but sadly you'll put the weight back on once you're being treated.

HEAT INTOLERANCE AND SWEATING

As metabolism is increased, your body produces excessive heat, which it then gets rid of by sweating. You won't enjoy warm weather or a centrally heated environment and may feel comfortable scantily dressed on a crisp winter's day. In extreme cases, your inability to tolerate heat may lead to disagreements with friends and colleagues, as you're constantly turning heating thermostats down, opening windows and tossing blankets or the duvet off the bed.

IRRITABILITY

This most often affects women with young families. You may find yourself increasingly unable to cope with the demands and stresses of looking after the children, you may lose your temper frequently and find that you're abnormally sensitive to criticism, bursting into tears for no apparent reason.

You may also find it difficult to concentrate, which can adversely affect your performance at school, college or in the workplace.

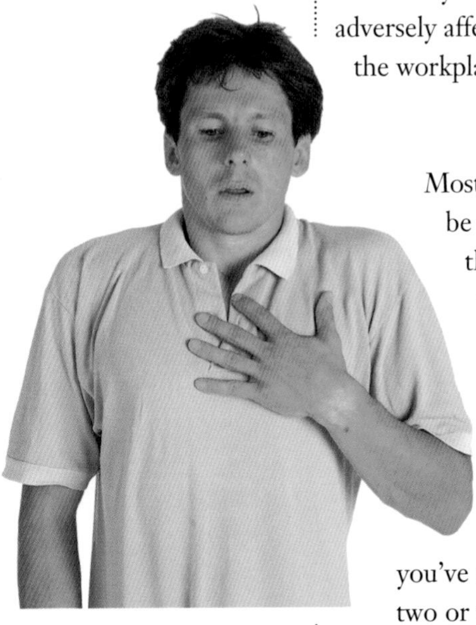

SHORTNESS OF BREATH
An overactive thyroid can make you feel breathless, which may be particularly apparent after physical exertion.

PALPITATIONS

Most patients experience palpitations, or you may be aware of your heart beating at a faster rate than normal. In severe, long-standing, untreated hyperthyroidism, particularly in more elderly people, there may be an irregular heartbeat, known as atrial fibrillation, and even heart failure.

BREATHLESSNESS

This is most likely to be noticeable when you've exerted yourself, for example after climbing two or three short flights of stairs. Individuals who already suffer from asthma may notice a worsening of their symptoms.

TREMOR

Most patients complain of shaky hands, which may be mistaken by friends and relatives for the tremor of alcoholism. You'll find it increasingly difficult to hold a cup still or insert a key into a lock, and your handwriting may deteriorate.

MUSCLE WEAKNESS

Characteristically, the thigh muscles become weak, making it hard to climb stairs or to get up from a squatting position or from a low chair without using your arms to help yourself up.

BOWEL MOVEMENT CHANGES

There tends to be an increase in their frequency such that you pass a softer than normal stool two or three times daily. Diarrhoea can occasionally be a problem.

IRREGULAR PERIODS

Periods are often irregular, light or even absent. Until the hyperthyroidism has been adequately treated, it may be difficult to conceive.

SKIN, HAIR AND NAIL PROBLEMS

You may find that your whole body itches, and people with Graves' disease, as mentioned earlier, may develop raised itchy patches on their lower legs and feet (pretibial myxoedema). Your hair will probably become thinner and finer than usual and won't take a perm very well. Your nails will be brittle and become rather unsightly.

EYE PROBLEMS

People with Graves' disease often have problems with their eyes. These include excessive watering made worse by wind and bright light, pain and grittiness as if there is sand in the eyes, double vision and blurring of vision. Many sufferers are also naturally upset because they develop exophthalmos (protruding eyes) as well as 'bags' under their eyes.

GOITRE

Although you will obviously be able to see when you have a goitre, it's unlikely to cause any actual symptoms other than a sensation that there is something in your neck that shouldn't be there.

HOW IS IT DIAGNOSED?

You will probably have had a blood test taken at your health centre or at the GP's surgery, but you may well have further blood tests done for confirmation when you go to the outpatients' clinic at the hospital. The specialist may also wish to carry out a thyroid scan to obtain more information about the cause of the hyperthyroidism as this may affect the type of treatment that you will need.

A thyroid scan requires a tiny dose of radioactive iodine or technetium, and this will be given either by mouth or by injection into a vein. The dose is so small that it can even be given to someone who is known to be allergic to iodine. Most specialists, however, would try to avoid radioactive scanning in a pregnant or breast-feeding woman.

After your GP has made the initial diagnosis, you'll probably have to wait before you can see the hospital specialist. In the meantime, your symptoms may be eased by taking one of the beta-blocker drugs such as propranolol, which counteracts to some extent the actions of thyroid hormones. This is most likely to be in a dose of 40 milligrams to be taken three or four times daily or in the form of propranolol (Inderal-LA) 160 milligrams daily as a single dose by mouth. Beta-blocking drugs should not be taken by people with asthma.

WHAT IS THE TREATMENT?

There are three forms of treatment for the hyperthyroidism caused by Graves' disease. These are drugs, surgery and radioactive iodine.

DRUGS

Antithyroid drugs are usually given to younger patients who go to their doctor when they have their first episode of hyperthyroidism. The most commonly used drug in the UK is carbimazole, which reduces the amount of hormones made by the thyroid gland. It is available as 5 milligram and 20 milligram tablets. A high dose (40–45 milligrams daily) is used initially, and your symptoms should start to improve after 10 to 14 days. Treatment is normally continued for 6–18 months, after which up to half the patients will have recovered and remain well. To start with, your specialist will review your treatment every four to six weeks, and the dose of carbimazole will be reduced in stages down to 5–15 milligrams daily in a single dose, depending upon the results of measurements of your blood levels of T3, T4 and TSH. Some specialists prefer to give a high dose of carbimazole throughout treatment, usually giving 40 milligrams daily, in the form of two 20 milligram tablets. If this high dose were to continue for several weeks or more, you would eventually develop an underactive thyroid gland, and therefore thyroxine is added to the carbimazole once thyroid hormone levels have returned to normal. The advantage of this type of treatment is that it doesn't need to be reviewed so often. It can also be particularly beneficial for patients with severe eye disease, but is not any more effective in controlling the symptoms of hyperthyroidism than carbimazole alone.

• **What you should know about drugs** Few people will experience any side effects from taking carbimazole, but those who do usually develop them within three to four weeks of starting treatment. A skin rash affects two per cent of patients, but the more serious reaction is a reduction in the number of white blood cells, which causes mouth ulcers and infection with a high fever. Your doctor should warn you about these possible effects when you first start the treatment. If you are affected, you should stop taking the drug and contact your GP straight away. You can then be given an alternative drug, called propylthiouracil, which works in a similar way to carbimazole.

SURGERY

Unfortunately, despite taking carbimazole or propylthiouracil alone or in combination with thyroxine for up to 18 months, about half of all patients will develop hyperthyroidism again and usually within two years of stopping the drug. If you're under 45 when you have your second bout of hyperthyroidism, it may be treated surgically by removing about three-quarters of your thyroid gland.

Before this operation can be done, however, it is necessary to restore thyroid hormone levels in your blood to normal with carbimazole. Once you've been given a date for the operation, you may be asked to take an iodine-containing medication for 10–14 days before surgery to reduce the size of the thyroid and its blood flow, which makes the job technically simpler for the surgeon. You'll usually go into hospital the day before your operation, which lasts about one hour, and you'll be allowed home between two and four days afterwards.

• **What you should know about surgery** The main disadvantage is that you will have a scar, but this usually becomes pale and unnoticeable among the skin creases in the neck. Alternatively you can wear jewellery or scarves to hide it. In very rare cases (less than one per cent), the parathyroid glands, which lie close to the thyroid and control the level of calcium in the blood, may be damaged, in which case long-term treatment with vitamin D capsules will be necessary. Equally rare is damage to one of the nerves supplying the voice box which may result in significant alteration to the quality of the voice. Although this wouldn't matter very much to most people, it could make surgery a less acceptable option to anyone who depends upon their voice for a living – an opera singer, for example.

In experienced hands, the initial results of surgery are good. Eighty per cent of sufferers will be cured immediately. However, 15 per cent will have had too much thyroid tissue removed and so will be hypothyroid, whereas five per cent will have had insufficient thyroid tissue removed and remain hyperthyroid. These failures are not the result of surgical incompetence, but have more to do with the nature of the underlying thyroid disease. What's more, over the passage of time, an increasing proportion of those patients whose hyperthyroidism was originally cured by surgery will develop an underactive thyroid gland. Recurrence of hyperthyroidism may even develop 20–40 years after apparently successful surgery. If the condition recurs, it is unusual to consider a second operation because surgery will be technically difficult and the risk of damage to surrounding structures increased.

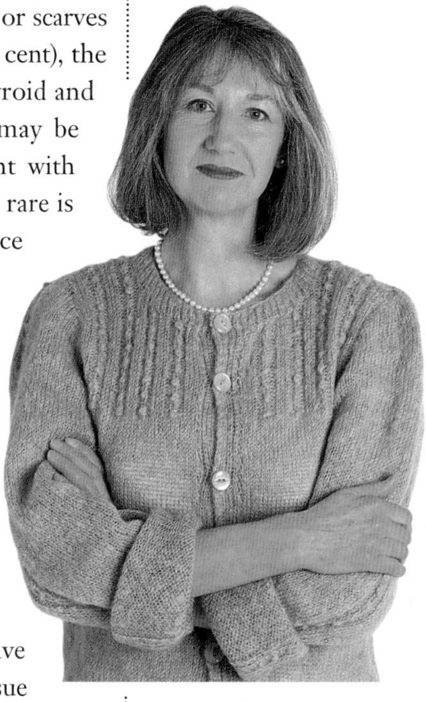

LITTLE TO SHOW
The scar left by thyroid surgery soon fades and becomes so indistinct that there is no need to cover the neck with scarves or jewellery.

Radioactive Iodine (Iodine-131)

Traditionally this form of treatment is reserved for patients aged over 40 or 45 and beyond child-bearing age or for younger individuals who have been sterilised.

This conservative approach was originally adopted because of concern that radioactive iodine might lead to any children conceived after treatment being born with abnormalities. In fact, there is no evidence for this, and in some hospitals there is a move towards using radioactive iodine in younger patients, as it is cheap and easy to administer.

Radioactive iodine is taken as a capsule or a drink that tastes like water, and is usually administered in hospital in a department of medical physics. Before receiving treatment, you may be asked to sign a consent form, and will have received instructions about avoiding places of entertainment and close contact with colleagues and young children for a period of a few days after therapy. Radioactive iodine is never prescribed for pregnant women, as it will adversely affect the fetal thyroid gland, and women are advised to avoid pregnancy for four months after treatment.

Radioactive iodine acts by destroying some of the thyroid cells and by preventing others from dividing, which is how they are normally replaced at the end of their lifespan. The treatment takes six to eight weeks to work and in the interim, depending upon the severity of the hyperthyroidism, you may be given propranolol or carbimazole to relieve your symptoms. You'll be asked to come back to hospital for a check-up in two to three months, and if you're one of the minority of people who is found to be still hyperthyroid, you'll be given a second dose of radioactive iodine.

Considering Which Treatment Is Right for You

An overactive thyroid may be treated with drugs, radioactive iodine or surgery. Choice of treatment depends on the individual patient concerned, and all options should be discussed with a specialist.

- No treatment is perfect, and you will need to discuss the options with your specialist. Some patients are not keen on surgery, even when a course of antithyroid drugs has been tried and failed.
- There is no reason why you shouldn't have a second, or even a third, course in the hope that the disease will ultimately 'burn itself out'. Indeed, before there was any form of treatment for the hyperthyroidism of Graves' disease, a proportion of patients got better spontaneously after months or years and then became hypothyroid.
- Some patients are unhappy at the prospect of radioactive iodine treatment, and some specialists consider that the best treatment for a young patient with severe hyperthyroidism and a large goitre is surgery.
- Whatever kind of treatment you have for hyperthyroidism, you will need regular follow-up, usually an annual blood test taken at a health centre or your GP's surgery.

• What you should know about radioactive iodine

The major problem with this treatment, however, is the development of hypothyroidism. This condition is most likely to appear in the first year after treatment, affecting about 50 per cent of people in some centres. In each year after that, around two to four per cent of people will be affected. It follows that the great majority become hypothyroid eventually, and it is essential that you should have regular check-ups either at the hospital or with your GP.

Once hypothyroidism has developed, treatment is with thyroxine, ultimately in a dose of 100 to 150 micrograms daily. There are no side-effects with thyroxine if the appropriate dose is taken regularly.

Case History 1: **HEART SYMPTOMS**

Although 70-year-old John Parry considered himself to be generally very healthy, he had recently noticed that his ankles were swelling. To start with, it was just at night, but then it happened all the time and his legs felt very heavy. One night at 1 a.m. he woke up gasping for breath and coughing up white frothy spit. His wife called an ambulance, and John was admitted to the local hospital within 20 minutes. The doctor on duty, Dr. Mackenzie, correctly diagnosed heart failure as the cause of the fluid accumulation in John's legs and lungs. He also noticed that John's pulse rate was very rapid and irregular, and an electrocardiogram showed this to be caused by atrial fibrillation. Mr. Parry was given oxygen using a facemask, an injection of a drug called frusemide (Lasix) to get rid of the excess fluid, and digoxin tablets to reduce the speed of his heart beat. As patients with atrial fibrillation are at risk of shedding blood clots from the heart, resulting in a stroke or a blocked artery in a leg, he was also given tablets called warfarin to thin the blood.

Dr. Mackenzie had at one time worked with an eminent endocrinologist and knew that atrial fibrillation could sometimes occur as a complication of an overactive thyroid gland, particularly in older patients.

Mr. Parry did indeed have hyperthyroidism, which turned out to be caused by Graves' disease, and he was treated with radioactive iodine. He was also given the antithyroid drug, carbimazole, for six weeks until the radioactive iodine had time to take effect.

Although to begin with Mr. Parry was concerned about the number of tablets he was taking when he left hospital, these had all been stopped within six months as his thyroid gland came under control. Even Mr. Parry's heart is now beating regularly and he is as fit as ever. His doctor carries out thyroid blood tests regularly to make sure that Mr. Parry is not developing an underactive thyroid gland as a result of the radioactive iodine treatment.

Case History 2: **RECURRENT SYMPTOMS**

Anna Robinson had had a previous episode of hyperthyroidism caused by Graves' disease in her mid-twenties, for which she had been given an 18-month course of carbimazole. At the age of 45, she noticed that she was troubled by the heat, but she put this symptom down to the 'change of life'.

However, when she began to lose weight and her hands became shaky, she realised that her thyroid gland was overactive again. At the local hospital the specialist suggested that she should be treated with radioactive iodine. In spite of reassurances and the evidence that this form of treatment was not associated with any risk other than the eventual onset of an underactive thyroid gland, Mrs. Robinson was uneasy.

She was aware of various articles in the newspapers suggesting a possible link between radiation and leukaemia in those living near to nuclear power stations, and she did not like the thought of having to avoid her new granddaughter, albeit only for a few days after treatment.

As she was a keen singer in the local church choir, thyroid surgery was felt not to be appropriate because of the possibility of a change in the quality of her voice.

Mrs. Robinson was relieved to learn there was no reason why she could not be treated with carbimazole again.

GRAVES' DISEASE AND THE EYES

The eye signs of Graves' disease (ophthalmopathy or orbitopathy) are present in most patients if the doctor looks hard enough. Sometimes these occur before the onset of the overactive thyroid gland or even for the first time after the successful treatment of the hyperthyroidism. One eye is often affected more than the other.

An early sign is retraction of the upper eyelid, which appears as if it has been pulled up, exposing more of the white of the eye and causing a staring appearance. This may improve after the raised levels of thyroid hormone have been restored to normal with treatment. Some patients complain of dry, gritty eyes, as if there is sand in them, and of constant blinking, others of excessive watering.

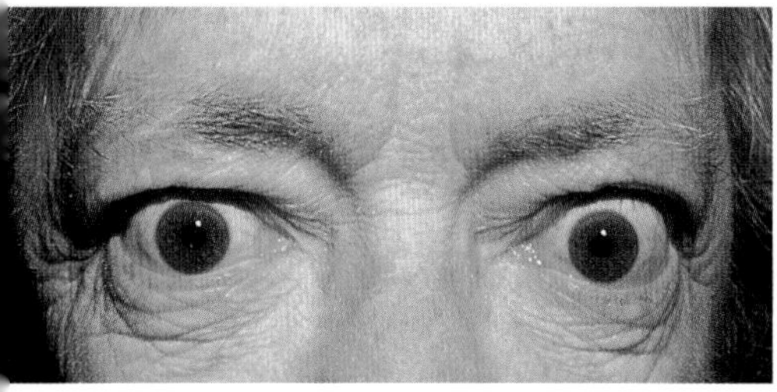

PROTRUDING EYES
Most patients with Graves' disease suffer some form of eye disorder. Bulging eyeballs, causing a staring appearance, are a common symptom.

The other features of thyroid eye disease result from a build-up of pressure behind the eyeball, which sits in a bony socket known as the orbit. The space between the eyeball and the back of the orbit contains the muscles that move the eye, the optic nerve, which relays messages to the brain, and fat.

In patients with thyroid eye disease, among other changes there is an accumulation of excessive amounts of water behind the eyeball, and the muscles and fat become swollen and boggy. The muscles increase in bulk two- or threefold and cease to work efficiently.

As a result, the normal movement of the eyes may be restricted and uncomfortable, with double vision (diplopia) and even the development of a squint. The increase in pressure behind the eyeballs pushes them forwards, producing the 'pop-eye' appearance known as exophthalmos or proptosis. The increased exposure of the

Rare Types of Hyperthyroidism

Occasionally, an overactive thyroid may be caused by a viral infection or by treatment with a particular drug.

- Mild hyperthyroidism, lasting for a few weeks, may occur after a viral infection of the thyroid; this is known as viral or de Quervain's thyroiditis, and the most prominent feature is severe pain and tenderness over the thyroid gland associated with symptoms of a flu-like illness. The hyperthyroidism rarely needs any treatment other than a beta-blocking drug, such as propranolol. There usually follows an equally short-lived period of mild hypothyroidism and then full recovery.
- The iodine-containing drug, amiodarone, which is used increasingly by heart specialists for the treatment of certain irregularities of heart rhythm, may cause hyperthyroidism.
  Your blood thyroid levels should be checked before you start taking the drug, and at six-monthly intervals while you're on it.

eyeballs makes them more prone to irritation from dust, grit, wind and sun, and the cornea may be damaged. In addition, some of the fat behind the eyeballs may be forced into the eyelids, contributing to their puffiness and the appearance of 'bags under the eyes'. Very rarely, in severely affected patients, the increased pressure may damage the optic nerve and cause partial or total loss of vision.

Treatment of the eye disease is not as satisfactory as that of the overactive thyroid gland. Smoking is thought to make it worse, as does poor control of the hyperthyroidism. It is very important, therefore, that you stop smoking completely and are careful to follow your doctor's instructions about dosage of tablets such as carbimazole or thyroxine. If you have dry eyes, you may find that a prescription for artificial tears helps, as it also does paradoxically for those with excessive watering. It may also be worth wearing dark glasses in sunny weather.

Patients with more advanced disease that threatens vision may need treatment with a steroid drug, such as prednisolone, which damps down the poorly understood processes leading to accumulation of water behind the eyeball. Alternatively, an operation may be required to remove part of the wall of the orbit, thereby reducing the pressure behind the eyeball.

Such a major undertaking is rarely necessary, however, and would be carried out only after close collaboration between thyroid and eye specialists. Most people who have Graves' disease find that their eye problems settle down considerably over a period of two to three years. At that stage, relatively minor surgery will correct double vision and reduce the 'staring' look and the bags under the eyes.

There is some evidence to suggest that the eye disease may deteriorate after treatment with radioactive iodine, and some specialists will not wish to prescribe this form of therapy for anyone whose eyes are badly affected. In some centres, radiotherapy has been used with some success in the treatment of thyroid eye disease.

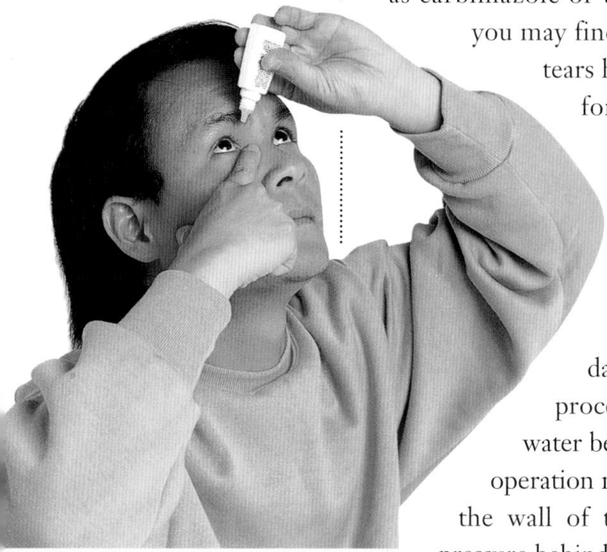

Eye Problems
You may find that artificial tears help if you suffer from dry or excessively watery eyes, a common complaint with thyroid disorders.

NODULAR GOITRE

This is treated either with surgery or with radioactive iodine. Unlike someone with Graves' disease, you're unlikely to develop hypothyroidism. It used to be fashionable after surgery to prescribe thyroxine to prevent regrowth of the goitre, which is common over a period of some 20 years, but this is not really useful unless you've developed hypothyroidism.

KEY POINTS

- Around three-quarters of cases of hyperthyroidism are caused by Graves' disease.
- Many people with Graves' disease may have inherited a tendency to develop it, although other factors are also involved in triggering the condition.
- The people most likely to develop Graves' disease are women between the ages of 40 and 50.
- Drugs, surgery and radioactive iodine are all possible ways of treating Graves' disease, but there is no single treatment that is right for everyone.
- Your specialists may want to discuss the treatment options with you before making the final decision on which approach is best for you.
- After treatment, you will need regular check-ups to ensure that you stay well.
- Most people with Graves' disease will experience some degree of eye problem, although they may only be minor irritations. More serious symptoms can be treated, and they usually settle over time.

Underactive thyroid

An underactive thyroid (hypothyroidism) occurs when the thyroid gland stops producing enough of the thyroid hormones, T3 and T4. In its most common form, affecting one per cent of the population (mainly middle-aged and elderly women), the thyroid gland shrinks as its cells are all destroyed by a subtle defect in the patient's immune system.

CHECKING THE THYROID
Your doctor will feel your thyroid gland to check its size and consistency.

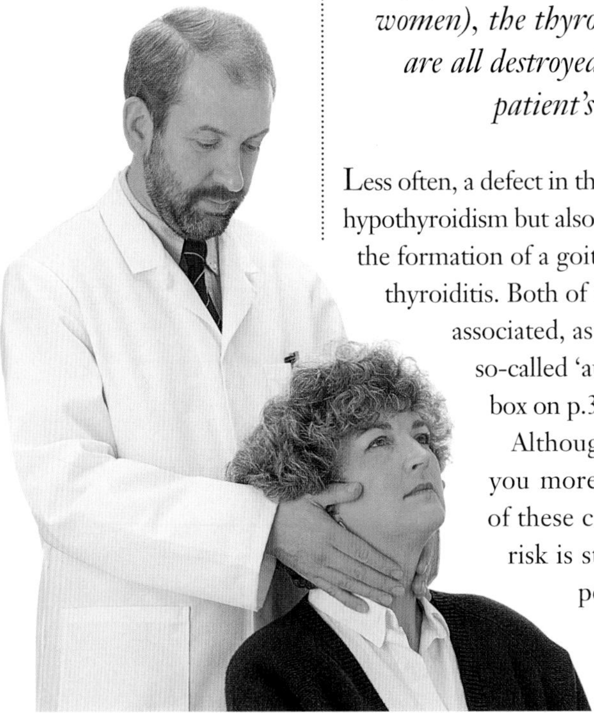

Less often, a defect in the immune system leads not only to hypothyroidism but also to enlargement of the thyroid and the formation of a goitre. This is known as Hashimoto's thyroiditis. Both of these types of hypothyroidism are associated, as is Graves' disease, with the other so-called 'autoimmune diseases' shown in the box on p.32.

Although having hypothyroidism makes you more likely to develop one or more of these conditions than other people, the risk is still small. The other reason why people develop hypothyroidism is as a result of the treatment of Graves' disease by surgery or with radioactive iodine.

HOW DOES IT DEVELOP?

Hypothyroidism does not come on overnight but slowly over many months, and you and your family may not notice the symptoms at first, or may simply put them down to ageing.

GPs now have ready access to the appropriate laboratory tests and, as a result, hypothyroidism is increasingly likely to be diagnosed at a relatively early stage when symptoms are mild. Hypothyroidism in its advanced state is sometimes known as 'myxoedema'.

It would be unusual to have all the symptoms mentioned below unless the diagnosis had been delayed for some reason for months or even years. You're more likely to go to your GP with rather vague complaints such as tiredness and weight gain, which could be due to a variety of causes.

You'll have a blood test and, if the result shows that you have low T4 and high TSH levels, this will be confirmation that you are suffering from hypothyroidism. Unless there is a complication, such as angina, you will be treated by your family doctor.

WHAT ARE THE SYMPTOMS?

Underactivity of the thyroid gland slows down the chemical reactions in the body, causing the following:

WEIGHT GAIN

Most patients gain from five to ten kilograms, although your appetite is normal or even less than usual.

SENSITIVITY TO THE COLD

You'll feel the cold very badly, and want to wear extra layers of clothing and sit close to the fire. You may well

Associated Diseases

Although the risk is small, an underactive thyroid can lead to an increased likelihood of developing one of the following auto-immune diseases:

- Pernicious anaemia: regular injections of vitamin B12 are necessary to maintain a normal blood count.
- Diabetes mellitus: a condition that usually requires treatment with insulin.
- Addison's disease: the adrenal glands, which sit on top of each kidney, produce insufficient cortisol and aldosterone, hormones that fortunately can be taken as tablets.
- Premature ovarian failure: this causes loss of periods, infertility and an early menopause.
- Underactivity of the parathyroid glands (glands adjacent to the thyroid): this leads to a low level of calcium in the blood, and to tetany, which is effectively treated with vitamin D capsules.
- Vitiligo: this is a skin disease in which there are areas of loss of pigmentation, giving a 'piebald' appearance.

suffer from muscle stiffness and spasm when you move suddenly, especially when it's cold.

MENTAL PROBLEMS

You may feel tired or sleepy, and slow down intellectually. Your reactions get slower but, fortunately, your sense of humour is unaffected. Older patients may be wrongly thought to be suffering from dementia, while some people experience depression and paranoia, which are the basis for what is popularly known as 'myxoedema madness'.

SLURRED SPEECH

Your voice becomes slow and husky and speech is often slurred.

HEART PROBLEMS

In contrast to a person with an overactive thyroid gland, your pulse rate is slow, at around 60 beats per minute. You may have high blood pressure, and an elderly patient with severe long-standing hypothyroidism is at risk of heart failure. Angina can be the first symptom of hypothyroidism.

CONSTIPATION

As the result of the general slowing down of the body's processes, you probably suffer from constipation.

Heavy Periods

Your periods become heavier (menorrhagia) if you haven't yet had your menopause.

Skin and Hair Problems

Your skin is likely to be rough and dry and to flake readily. It tends to be pale and your eyelids, hands and feet swell. Some people may find their skin has a lemon-yellowish tint, and prominent blood vessels in the cheeks add a purplish flush. Sitting too close to the fire can cause a 'granny's tartan' to appear on the skin of your legs. Some people get the skin condition known as vitiligo. Your hair becomes dry and brittle and the outer part of your eyebrows may be missing.

Nervous System Disorders

You may become a little deaf and have trouble with your balance. If your fingers tingle, especially during the night, shaking your hands vigorously should relieve it.

What Is the Treatment?

Treatment is with thyroxine, which is available in the UK as 25, 50 and 100 microgram tablets. Normally, thyroxine treatment is begun slowly and you'll be prescribed a daily dose of 50 micrograms for three to four weeks, increasing to 100 micrograms daily for a further three to four weeks and then to 150 micrograms daily. You'll then have another blood test some three months after starting treatment to assess whether any further minor adjustment of dose is necessary. The aim is to restore levels of T4 and TSH in the blood to normal.

You should start to feel better within two to three weeks; you'll lose weight and notice the puffiness around your eyes disappearing quite soon, but your skin and hair texture may take three to six months to recover fully. Normally you'll have to expect to stay on thyroxine treatment for life.

Case History: **SUDDEN FALL IN GLUCOSE LEVELS**

Jean Spencer was 17 and in her final year at school, hoping to go to university to study law. She had had diabetes since she was 11 and gave herself insulin injections twice each day. Control of her diabetes had always been very satisfactory and her dose of insulin did not vary much. She had been puzzled, however, for the last three months because she did not seem to require as much insulin as before. On four occasions she had almost become unconscious in class because of a low level of glucose in her blood but had been brought round with sugary drinks by her teacher.

Once she did not respond, and she was rushed to hospital, given a glucose drip into a vein and kept in overnight. Jean's parents and her teacher were also concerned because she was not concentrating in class and her results in the mock exams had not been nearly as good as expected. She had also begun to complain of the cold and had not been able to sing in the school Christmas Concert because her voice had become husky. It was her aunt, visiting from Canada, who recognised the change in Jean's appearance since her last visit the previous year.

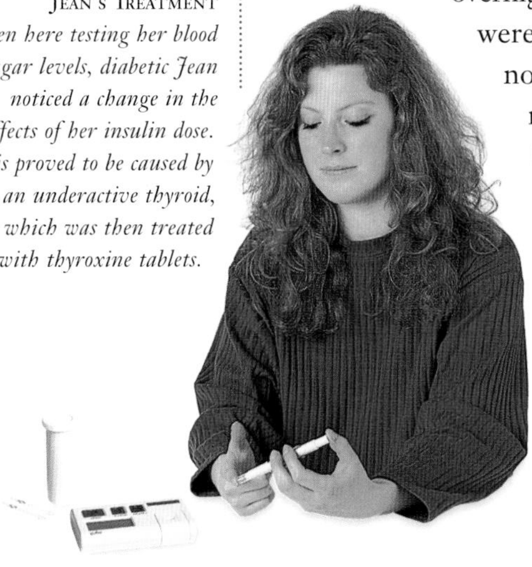

JEAN'S TREATMENT
Seen here testing her blood sugar levels, diabetic Jean noticed a change in the effects of her insulin dose. This proved to be caused by an underactive thyroid, which was then treated with thyroxine tablets.

She herself had developed an underactive thyroid gland 10 years earlier and suggested to Jean that she have a blood test. Jean is now taking thyroxine tablets, like her aunt, and her insulin dose has returned to its previous level. She passed her A levels with flying colours and is now in her first term at university studying law.

SPECIAL SITUATIONS

The level of various fats or lipids in the blood is increased in hypothyroidism, and in people who have had the condition unrecognised for a long time, the coronary arteries become narrowed by fatty deposits. Insufficient blood reaches the heart muscle, especially during exercise, and the sufferer will get pain in the middle of their chest, a symptom of angina.

Treatment with thyroxine may worsen the angina and someone with this problem will be started on a lower dose and have it increased more slowly than normal. It may be necessary to have an operation to improve the blood flow through the coronary arteries before or after starting thyroxine treatment. Thyroxine dosage should also be carefully monitored during pregnancy (see p.38).

TEMPORARY HYPOTHYROIDISM

It is usually necessary for treatment with thyroxine to be continued throughout the patient's life. However, if you develop hypothyroidism in the first three to four months after surgery or radioactive iodine treatment for Graves' disease it may be short-lived, lasting only a few weeks, and you may not need any treatment. The same is true for the hypothyroidism that occurs as a complication of postpartum thyroiditis (see p.43) or de Quervain's thyroiditis (see p.27).

MILD HYPOTHYROIDISM

Most GPs will arrange for someone to have a blood test even when they only suspect thyroid problems. Quite minor abnormalities are often picked up in patients who visit their doctor because of a variety of rather vague symptoms, such as tiredness, or in people who have a family history of autoimmune disease.

The most common finding is the combination of a 'normal' T4 but raised TSH level, known among doctors as subclinical hypothyroidism. It is known that around five to 20 per cent of these people will develop more obvious hypothyroidism in each following year. For this reason, it is now common practice to 'nip things in the bud' by prescribing thyroxine when the abnormality has been found on more than one occasion. This may not have any dramatic effect on the individual concerned, but preventive medicine is better than cure.

DRUG-RELATED PROBLEMS

Lithium carbonate, which is widely used for depression and mania, may cause goitre and hypothyroidism. When, as normally happens, a person needs to keep taking lithium carbonate, continued treatment with thyroxine will be necessary.

Amiodarone, which is used in the treatment of certain heart irregularities, may not only cause hyperthyroidism but also hypothyroidism, and anyone who is taking it will need thyroid blood tests from time to time.

KEY POINTS

- Hypothyroidism usually comes on slowly, and your symptoms are likely to be vague at first.
- Your GP will be able to confirm the diagnosis with a simple blood test.
- Treatment is with tablets, which you will probably need to take for the rest of your life.
- Some people who have been hypothyroid for many years may suffer from chest pain caused by angina and, because thyroxine aggravates the problem, their dosage will need careful monitoring. If you already have angina when your thyroid condition is first discovered, your treatment will be adjusted to take account of this.
- If your thyroid blood test is only slightly abnormal, you may be given preventive treatment with thyroxine.

Thyroid disease and pregnancy

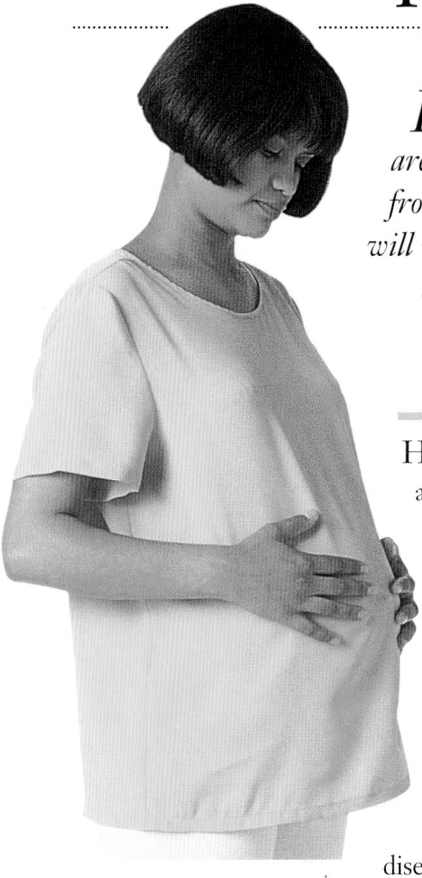

It is important to tell your doctor that you are planning to become pregnant if you suffer from any kind of thyroid disease. Your doctor will want to keep your thyroid hormones under careful control through the pregnancy to prevent any harm to the baby.

GRAVES' DISEASE

Hyperthyroidism occurring during pregnancy is almost always the result of Graves' disease. It is not a common event, however, as autoimmune diseases, of which Graves' disease is an example, tend to improve of their own accord during pregnancy. Also, women with an overactive thyroid gland are relatively infertile because a greater proportion of their menstrual cycles do not release an egg from the ovaries.

As the thyroid-stimulating antibody that is responsible for the hyperthyroidism of Graves' disease crosses the placenta and passes from the blood of the mother to that of the developing child, it too will have an overactive thyroid gland like its mother. Fortunately, the antithyroid drugs also cross the placenta and good control of hyperthyroidism in the mother will

DRUGS AND PREGNANCY
Close control of the activity of the thyroid gland is important during pregnancy.

ensure that the fetus comes to no harm. Failure to recognise hyperthyroidism or to treat it adequately in a pregnant woman may lead to miscarriage, and overtreatment with antithyroid drugs may lead to goitre developing in the fetus.

It is important, therefore, that the patient is prescribed the lowest dose of carbimazole possible to restore thyroid hormone levels in the blood to normal, and these levels are checked every four to six weeks, in close cooperation with the obstetrician who is caring for her. The carbimazole is usually stopped four weeks before the expected date of delivery to make sure that there is no possibility of the fetus being hypothyroid at a crucial time in its development.

If hyperthyroidism recurs in the mother after the baby is born, and she is breast-feeding, she will be treated with propylthiouracil rather than carbimazole because it is excreted in the milk much less and will not therefore affect the baby.

There are some reports from North America that carbimazole is associated with a rare disease in the newborn baby, known as aplasia cutis, in which there is a defect in the skin covering a small part of the scalp. The view in the UK is, however, that the risk has been overestimated, if it is present at all. Most specialists in this country are happy to prescribe carbimazole during pregnancy. Some, however, may prefer to use propylthiouracil and to change from carbimazole before conception, if possible. The dose of propylthiouracil is ten times that of carbimazole, and it is available as 50 milligram tablets only.

Radioactive iodine treatment is never given during pregnancy. Surgery is occasionally advised round week 20 of pregnancy for patients who develop side-effects to the drugs or who take them irregularly, thereby putting the fetus at risk.

Hyperthyroidism in The Newborn

In most women with Graves' disease, during pregnancy the thyroid stimulating antibody disappears or its level in the blood becomes low. In some, however, the level remains high, and as blood from the mother is in contact with that of the fetus throughout pregnancy these high levels are also present in the blood of the newborn and may cause hyperthyroidism. It is possible to predict those babies most likely to develop hyperthyroidism by finding high levels of antibodies in the mother's blood towards the end of pregnancy. Hyperthyroidism in the newborn, if detected at this stage, is easily treated and lasts only 2–3 weeks until the antibody from the mother is broken down and inactivated. Very occasionally, mothers who have been treated successfully for Graves' disease in the past continue to produce thyroid stimulating antibody and their newborn offspring are at risk of developing hyperthyroidism.

All newborn babies in the UK have a blood test shortly after birth to detect any deficiency of thyroid hormone, a quite separate condition (see p.42).

Case History 1: **CONCEPTION AND PREGNANCY**

Rebecca and her husband had been trying to have a second child for three years without success. Rebecca had conceived twice but, unfortunately, on each occasion had miscarried at about ten weeks. She felt and looked well and, although she had lost a few pounds in weight, she put this down to her busy lifestyle of running the home, looking after an active five-year-old son, and working part-time as a secretary. She was a little anxious that her periods, which used to be as regular as clockwork, had become much lighter and, on occasion, were missed.

During her weekly telephone call to her mother, she learned that her cousin in Australia had recently been diagnosed as having an overactive thyroid gland. She consulted her GP and, despite her lack of obvious signs (having neither a goitre nor bulging eyes), tests on a sample of her blood showed the presence of mild hyperthyroidism, and this was confirmed at the local hospital as being caused by Graves' disease. Treatment was started with carbimazole, initially in a dose of 30 milligrams daily and, after five months of treatment, Rebecca was pregnant.

She was reviewed by the endocrinologist every four weeks and, by the middle of her pregnancy, she needed to take only 5 milligrams of carbimazole every day. The drug was stopped four weeks before the expected date of delivery and she gave birth to a healthy girl whose heel-prick blood test at seven days was normal, with no evidence of thyroid abnormality. Rebecca breast-fed her daughter but, after four months, developed hyperthyroidism, again as a result of Graves' disease because the thyroid-stimulating antibody was present in her blood. She decided to change to bottle-feeding and her hyperthyroidism was then treated with carbimazole as before. Had she opted to continue breast-feeding, propylthiouracil would have been prescribed instead.

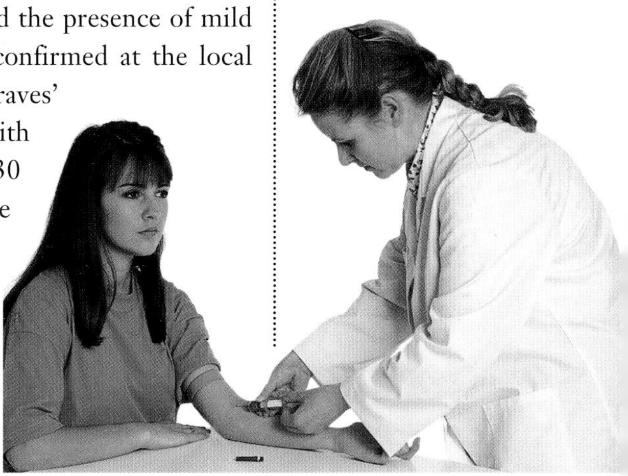

Taking a Sample
In Rebecca's case, blood tests showed that she was suffering from mild hyperthyroidism, which was increasing her chances of having a miscarriage.

HYPOTHYROIDISM

Most patients with hypothyroidism are already taking thyroxine when they become pregnant. Although mild hypothyroidism is unlikely to reduce fertility, patients with severe thyroid deficiency of prolonged duration are unlikely to become pregnant or, if they conceive, to maintain their pregnancy.

The dose of thyroxine may need to be increased during pregnancy by as much as 50 micrograms daily. Blood tests will be taken every three months to check whether the dose needs to be increased. The dose before pregnancy can be taken once again three to four weeks after childbirth. The thyroid gland of the fetus develops independently of the mother and makes its own thyroid hormones. The baby will therefore not be at risk if you forget the occasional dose of thyroxine, but making a habit of not taking it increases the chances of miscarriage.

HYPOTHYROIDISM IN THE NEWBORN

HYPOTHYROIDISM IN BABIES
A simple pin prick test on the heel is performed on all newborn babies. This is used to test for hypothyroidism.

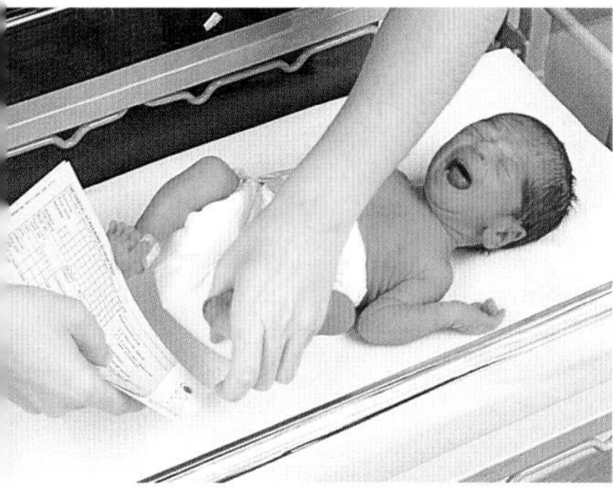

One in about 3,500 newborn babies has an underactive thyroid gland as a result of failure of the gland to develop normally. In the past, the problem was not recognised until the child was several weeks old, by which time he or she would have been likely to develop permanent mental and physical handicap – the condition known then as cretinism. Today, however, all newborn babies are screened by a blood test for hypothyroidism between five and seven days after they are born. Any affected children are given prompt treatment that ensures that they develop normally. Treatment is usually for life, but in a few babies the hypothyroidism is temporary. Temporary hypothyrodism is a result of being born to a mother with an underactive thyroid gland, in whom there are blocking antibodies that cross the placenta and have the opposite effect of the stimulating antibodies that produce Graves' disease, and neonatal hyperthyroidism (see p.40).

AFTER CHILDBIRTH

Although the hyperthyroidism of Graves' disease tends to get better on its own during pregnancy, it often returns in a severe form within a few months of delivery. There is, however, another form of hyperthyroidism that may develop in the first year after childbirth, almost always in patients who have underlying autoimmune thyroid disease such as Hashimoto's thyroiditis, which may not have been recognised previously. The hyperthyroidism is mild, lasts only a few weeks and can be treated with a beta-blocker if necessary. This phase may be followed by an equally transient episode of mild hypothyroidism not requiring treatment, and then usually followed by full recovery. A similar pattern may occur in future pregnancies and many patients ultimately develop a permanently underactive thyroid. It is important to distinguish between what is known as postpartum thyroiditis, not requiring treatment, and Graves' disease, which does. To do so, it may be necessary to measure the concentration of the thyroid-stimulating antibody in the blood, which is usually present in Graves' disease, or the ability of the thyroid gland to concentrate radioactive iodine or technetium, which is lacking in postpartum thyroiditis. Postpartum thyroiditis affects about five per cent of women but most patients do not complain of symptoms. There does not appear to be any association between the thyroid blood test abnormalities and postnatal depression.

Case History 2: **POSTPARTUM THYROIDITIS**

Flora Stewart was 25 and happily married to her lawyer husband, William, and they'd had their first child, Jane, five months earlier. Their relationship began to deteriorate when Flora became weepy and short-tempered, snapping at William for no good reason.

Flora was also sleeping badly and William noticed that Flora's hands sometimes trembled. However, they both put all this down to hormonal changes following her pregnancy and the birth of their baby, and assumed that before long everything would be back to normal.

However, when Flora began to complain of palpitations William persuaded her to visit their GP. The doctor thought that Flora might have an overactive thyroid gland and his suspicions were confirmed by a blood test.

On hearing the news Flora was concerned, because her mother had suffered from Graves' disease when she was in her thirties and her eyes were still very prominent 20 years later, even though the hyperthyroidism had been cured. In order to relieve some of Flora's symptoms, her GP prescribed a long-acting form of propranolol (Inderal LA) 80 milligrams, to be taken once daily. He also suggested that Flora should see a specialist at the local hospital. By the time her appointment came round four weeks later, Flora felt much better and a repeat blood sample showed that her thyroid gland had become very slightly underactive. The diagnosis was not that of Graves' disease, but postpartum thyroiditis, and Flora was reassured that she would not get bulging eyes like her mother. The propranolol was stopped, and another blood test two months later was entirely normal.

Flora now knows that she may get the symptoms of postpartum thyroiditis after further pregnancies, and that she has an increased chance of developing a permanently underactive thyroid gland at some stage in the future.

However, her GP will do a thyroid blood test every year to make sure that it is detected before she can develop severe symptoms.

KEY POINTS

- If you are planning a baby, tell your doctor as you may need to change to a different drug.
- Your doctor will keep a close watch on you during pregnancy, but your treatment will not harm your developing baby.
- Some women will develop mild thyroid disease after having a baby, but this is easily treated. If you are experiencing similar symptoms to those described in Flora's story on p.44, it is worth asking your GP whether this could be the cause.
- Although your child may be born with hypothyroidism if you suffer from it, like all newborns he or she will be given a routine test shortly after birth and treated if necessary.

Enlarged thyroid

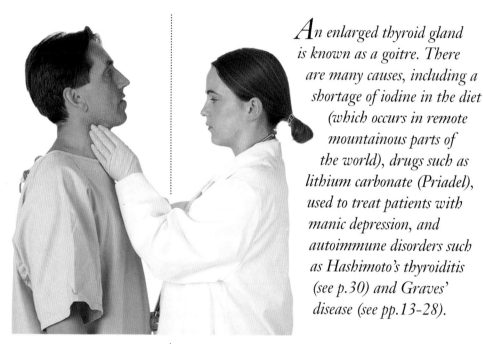

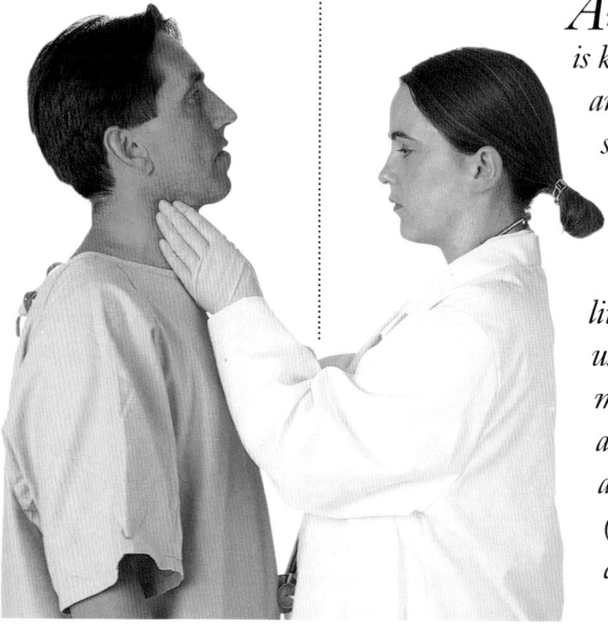

An enlarged thyroid gland is known as a goitre. There are many causes, including a shortage of iodine in the diet (which occurs in remote mountainous parts of the world), drugs such as lithium carbonate (Priadel), used to treat patients with manic depression, and autoimmune disorders such as Hashimoto's thyroiditis (see p.30) and Graves' disease (see pp.13-28).

ASSESSING THE THYROID
Your doctor will usually be able to confirm the presence of a goitre by feeling your neck.

The cause of most goitres in the UK is not known. Such goitres are called 'simple goitres', despite the fact that there are almost certainly complex reasons for their development. Although the thyroid gland is enlarged, it continues to produce normal amounts of hormones and the patient is referred to as 'euthyroid' as opposed to hyperthyroid or hypothyroid. At first, in teenagers and young adults, the goitre is evenly or diffusely enlarged. During the next 15 to 25 years, whatever caused the thyroid to grow abnormally in the first place remains and it continues to grow but becomes full of lumps or nodules. By the time the young person reaches middle age, the goitre will have become lumpy, when it is known medically as a 'multinodular goitre'.

SIMPLE DIFFUSE GOITRE

Most of those who have a simple diffuse goitre are young women between the ages of 15 and 25. If you are one of them, you (or your relatives) will have noticed a symmetrical, smooth swelling in the front of your neck. You may have had it for some years but thought it was just 'puppy fat'. The goitre will move up and down when you swallow. It is not tender, however, and does not usually cause difficulty in swallowing but you may experience a tight sensation in your neck. The goitre may vary slightly in size and be more noticeable at the time of a period or during pregnancy. It isn't normally a problem appearance-wise – quite the opposite as far as some people are concerned. For example, the great seventeenth and eighteenth century artists often added a goitre to the female figure to enhance her beauty!

HOW IS IT DIAGNOSED?

Usually your GP will want you to be seen by a specialist to exclude rarer causes of goitre. The specialist can normally do this by feeling your neck and by taking blood tests.

WHAT IS THE TREATMENT?

No treatment is necessary for simple diffuse goitre. In the past, iodine (often added to milk) or thyroxine tablets were given but neither is effective. Many people find that their goitre becomes less noticeable or even disappears over a period of two to three years.

SIMPLE MULTINODULAR GOITRE

If you are middle-aged, you will probably become aware of a swelling in your neck while washing or applying make-up in front of a mirror. In fact, the goitre will have been present for many years but has now reached a critical size or it may be that your neck has become thinner. The goitre is often more obvious on one side of the neck than the other. It may vary in size from being barely visible to other people to so large that you feel you have to hide it by wearing scarves or high-necked sweaters. A few people notice the enlarged thyroid gland for the first time because internal bleeding causes increased swelling which is accompanied by discomfort in the neck, like a bruise, lasting a few days.

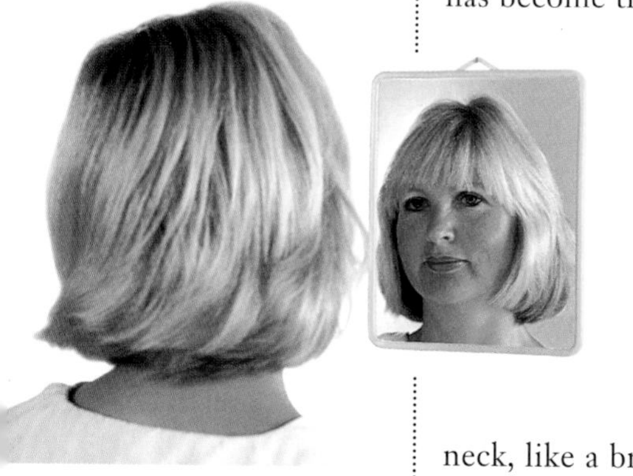

BECOMING AWARE
Many people first notice that they have developed a goitre when looking in the mirror.

If the goitre is large there may be difficulty in swallowing dry, solid food and, if the trachea (windpipe) is squashed to any extent, there may be difficulty in breathing. Singers, in particular, will notice a change in their voice.

HOW IS IT DIAGNOSED?

Your GP may take a blood sample to check that your thyroid hormone levels are normal but will usually ask a specialist for advice about further investigations and treatment.

The specialist may wish to carry out one or more of the following tests:

- **X-rays and breathing tests** These will reveal whether the goitre is compressing or squashing the trachea (the windpipe).

- **Ultrasound scan** A probe, the size of a small hand torch, is passed over the skin of the front of the neck and an image of the goitre is formed on a TV screen. As well as showing its size and extent, it will also highlight any cysts or nodules that the specialist may not have noticed when examining the neck.
- **Isotope scan** This technique provides a different type of image, which shows whether the nodules in the goitre are likely to be producing thyroid hormones, in which case the development of an overactive thyroid is more likely in future years. It is obtained by injecting a tiny amount of radioactive substance called technetium-99m into a vein. About half an hour after the injection you lie under a sophisticated form of camera for a few minutes.
- **Fine needle aspiration** This involves attaching a needle of the same size as that used for taking a blood sample to the end of a syringe, then, while you're lying down, passing it without local anaesthetic through the skin of the neck into the enlarged thyroid gland. The discomfort is no more than that felt during a straightforward blood test. By pulling on the plunger and moving the needle up and down a tiny distance within the goitre, the doctor can obtain thyroid cells for analysis. These are smeared on to a glass slide and, after processing in the pathology laboratory, are examined under a microscope. The appearance of the cells will help to determine whether the thyroid enlargement is the result of a malignant tumour.

FINE NEEDLE ASPIRATION
In this test, a needle is inserted into the thyroid gland to extract a sample of thyroid cells for analysis.

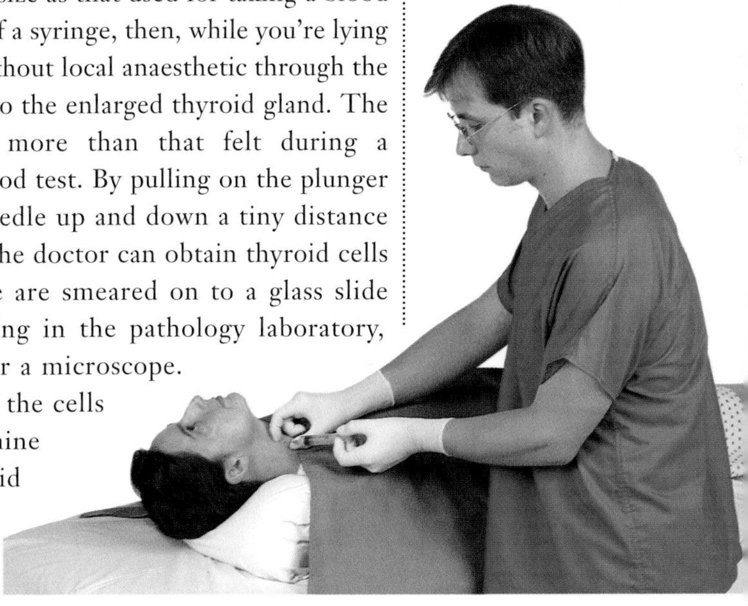

Fine needle aspiration, commonly known as FNA, is not often carried out in patients with a multinodular goitre unless the gland is very much bigger on one side than the other, or the goitre is growing very rapidly.

WHAT IS THE TREATMENT?

If your goitre is relatively small, you probably won't need any treatment. Your GP will check thyroid hormone levels in your blood every one to two years as there is a possibility of the gland becoming overactive and causing hyperthyroidism at some stage during the next 20 years or so. Although thyroxine tablets are prescribed in certain parts of the world in an attempt to shrink the goitre, they are of little or no benefit and may cause hyperthyroidism.

If the goitre becomes so large that it looks really unattractive or is compressing the windpipe, the most effective treatment is an operation to remove most of the thyroid gland.

No treatment is necessary before surgery and you will be in hospital for about three days. The complications are the same as those for surgery for Graves' disease (see p.21). You may need thyroxine treatment afterwards as there may be insufficient thyroid tissue left to produce adequate amounts of hormones.

In patients who aren't fit enough for surgery or who don't want to have an operation, it may be possible to reduce the size of the goitre by about 50 per cent by giving radioactive iodine. A large dose is necessary, and you may have to be admitted to hospital for 24 – 48 hours. If so, you'll be given a single room to avoid contaminating other patients or visitors with radioactivity. It may take several months for the goitre to shrink. It is unlikely that the thyroid will become underactive. This is because the radioactive iodine is mainly concentrated within the nodules and, as they become smaller, the thyroid tissue surrounding them that has been dormant and unaffected by the radiation wakes up and starts to produce thyroid hormones.

Case History: OVERACTIVE THYROID GLAND

Jenny Morris was a single woman in her seventies who had been an accomplished actress. She always wore a silk scarf around her neck, day and night, summer and winter. Friends and neighbours thought it was part of her slightly eccentric personality, but when Jenny was admitted to hospital as an emergency with abdominal pain due to gallstones, the scarf was removed to reveal a large goitre and a scar from a previous thyroid operation.

Miss Morris explained that the operation had been carried out for a goitre when she was quite young. In her mid-forties the goitre had appeared again, but she had been told that further surgery was out of the question because a second operation would be technically more difficult and any damage to the nearby nerve supply to the voice box (larynx) would ruin her stage career. As time passed the goitre had gradually grown and grown, and she had taken to wearing the scarves to avoid embarrassment.

Blood tests in hospital showed her to have a slightly overactive thyroid gland, and three months after treatment with radioactive iodine her blood test came back to normal. Equally important, a year later, the size of the goitre had been reduced by at least a half, and she happily abandoned her scarves!

THYROID NODULES

Single lumps or nodules in the thyroid are common, and can occur at any age. Women are more likely to be affected than men.

A single thyroid nodule varies in size from that of a pea to a golf ball or even larger. Like a goitre, the nodule is usually discovered by accident while you're washing or looking in a mirror. Bleeding into the nodule may cause pain which alerts you to its presence. Alternatively, the nodule may be discovered during a medical examination for some quite unrelated problem, although neither you nor your family had noticed it before. Most women are aware of the significance of a lump in the breast, and so naturally suspect that a nodule in the thyroid may also mean cancer.

This is why your GP will probably want you to see a specialist. In fact, the great majority of single thyroid nodules are not cancers of the thyroid.

HOW IS IT DIAGNOSED?

If you have a single thyroid nodule, your blood test will show normal levels of T3, T4 and TSH, which means you're classified medically as 'euthyroid'; the exception is the 'toxic adenoma' in which the thyroid blood tests will demonstrate an overactive thyroid gland. The thyroid specialist will wish to examine your neck carefully as about half of all patients thought to have a single nodule are in fact found to have generalised nodular enlargement of the thyroid known as multinodular goitre. In this case you can be assured that your condition is not serious.

People who need further investigations may have an X ray, ultrasound or radioisotope scan of their thyroid, but the single most important test is fine needle aspiration (FNA) of the lump. The technique is simple, quick and, if necessary, can be carried out two or three times as it doesn't cause pain or undue discomfort. FNA is one of the most important advances in the care of people with thyroid disease. In the past the majority of those with a single thyroid nodule had to have surgery, but many operations can now be avoided simply by examining a small sample of thyroid cells obtained by aspiration in the outpatient clinic. The outcome of the FNA will be one of those indicated in the box below.

Benign (non-cancerous) nodules may continue to enlarge over many years and eventually may get so big that an

What Does Fine Needle Aspiration Reveal?

Fine needle aspiration, in which a few thyroid cells are removed for examination, is used to investigate thyroid nodules. The outcome will be one of the following:

- The needle will remove fluid and the nodule will disappear: this means that the nodule must have been a thyroid cyst and no further treatment is needed. Should the cyst recur it can be aspirated again, but you will need an operation to remove that half of the thyroid containing the cyst if it comes back yet again.
- The cells removed from the nodule show that it is a benign lump and therefore you don't have cancer. Unless the swelling is sufficiently large to be disfiguring, when surgery would be necessary, you can be reassured that no treatment is needed.
- The cells removed are malignant, which means that the nodule is thyroid cancer, and you will need an immediate operation.
- Sometimes, because of the small number of cells removed, it may be impossible to be certain whether the nodule is benign or malignant. You will need an operation to remove the entire nodule so that it can be examined carefully under the microscope.

operation is needed to remove them for the sake of your appearance. If you are worried that the lump is harbouring a cancer, your specialist may suggest operating to remove the nodule so that it can be examined microscopically and the question resolved once and for all.

KEY POINTS

- In non-iodine deficient countries, the cause of a goitre usually remains a mystery.
- Young people with a simple diffuse goitre rarely need any treatment.
- You will probably be referred to a specialist to have a multinodular goitre investigated, and may have several tests.
- A small goitre may be left alone, but you will have regular blood tests done by your GP as there is a chance of developing hyperthyroidism later on.
- An operation or treatment with radioactive iodine may be necessary if a goitre is causing problems.
- Thyroxine tablets won't help to shrink a goitre, although they are still prescribed in some other countries.
- Although people who develop thyroid nodules often worry that the lump may be cancer, this rarely turns out to be the case.
- The simple and painless investigation known as fine needle aspiration means that far fewer people now have to have surgery.
- If you're concerned about your appearance or can't stop worrying about the possibility of cancer, you can have an operation to remove the nodule.

Cancer of the thyroid gland

Malignant tumours of the thyroid gland are rare. For example, a specialist may see 50 to 100 patients with hyperthyroidism caused by Graves' disease for every one with thyroid cancer.

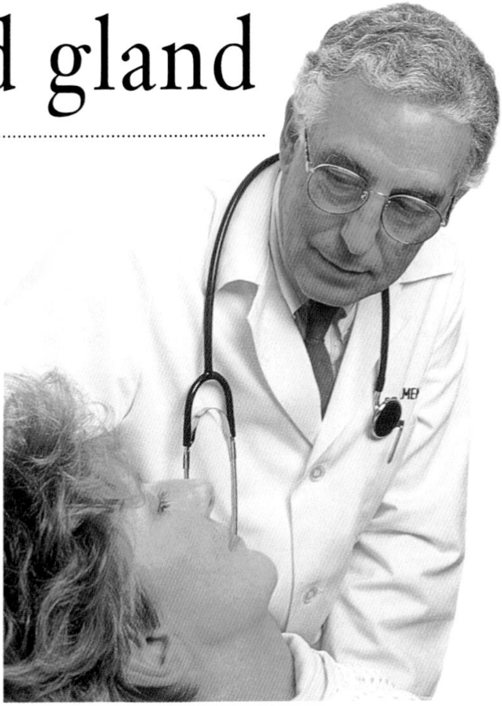

CONFIRMING THE DIAGNOSIS
Your doctor will examine any lumps in your neck, but any diagnosis of thyroid cancer can only be made in hospital after fine needle aspiration or surgery.

The two types of thyroid cancer that doctors see most often are:

- Papillary cancer, which mostly affects young women and children.
- Follicular cancer, which is unusual before the age of 30.

These medical terms describe the appearance of the tumour under the microscope. In papillary cancer, the tumour contains papillae or fronds, whereas in follicular cancer, although the appearance is distinctly abnormal, there are still structures that resemble the normal follicles of the thyroid. Both cancers can occur at any age, however. Provided diagnosis and treatment are at an early stage, the person may have a normal lifespan; in other words, you're still more likely to die of a stroke or a heart attack in old age.

HOW IS IT DIAGNOSED?

Most patients visit their GP with a lump in the neck or because of rapid growth of a goitre which they've had for many years. The diagnosis of thyroid cancer is made at a hospital visit by fine needle aspiration or following surgery.

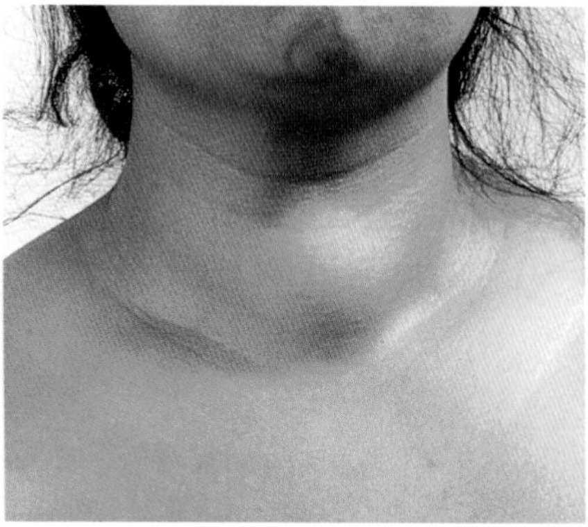

CANCER OF THE THYROID
The first sign of thyroid cancer is a painless nodule in the neck, in or near the thyroid gland.

Occasionally, the patient consults their doctor because of enlarged lymph nodes in the neck which may at first be thought to be caused by Hodgkin's disease. However, a biopsy will show that the patient actually has papillary cancer which has spread from the thyroid gland via the lymphatic system to the nearby lymph nodes.

WHAT IS THE TREATMENT?

Thyroid cancer is normally treated by complete or partial removal of the thyroid gland. Radioactive iodine is commonly used postoperatively to kill any remaining cancerous cells.

SURGERY

Papillary cancer is usually treated by removal of as much of the thyroid gland as possible (total thyroidectomy) because there is a tendency for the cancer to occur in various places throughout the gland. Any large lymph nodes containing the cancer are also removed at this stage. In contrast, follicular cancer usually develops in only one part of the thyroid and removal of half of the gland (hemithyroidectomy) is all that may be necessary.

No special treatment is required before the operation and you can usually go home after three days.

Radioactive Iodine

It is not possible to remove every last part of the thyroid gland by means of surgery and some patients with papillary cancer will be given a large dose of radioactive iodine (iodine-131) to kill any remaining cells. The radioactive iodine is given as a liquid or a capsule in hospital. You will have to stay in hospital for 24 – 48 hours, in a single room, separated from the other patients to avoid contaminating them with radioactivity.

The radioactive iodine is usually given three to four weeks after your operation and before thyroxine tablets have been started, as it is most effective when the patient is hypothyroid and TSH levels in the blood are high. If for some reason you have already started taking thyroxine to prevent you from becoming hypothyroid after removal of your thyroid gland, you will be taken off the treatment some four weeks before being given radioactive iodine.

Towards the end of the period without thyroxine you may feel tired but will come to no harm. Very recently it has become possible to increase the level of TSH in the blood by giving injections of synthetic TSH (thyrogen), identical to that made by the human pituitary gland, avoiding the need to stop thyroxine.

Radioactive iodine is not given so often postoperatively to patients with a follicular cancer.

Thyroxine

Doctors believe that the rate of growth of papillary and follicular cancers of the thyroid may be increased by the hormone TSH. An important part of the treatment, therefore, is to make sure that you take enough thyroxine to ensure that the level of TSH in your blood becomes undetectable. Patients with thyroid cancer need a slightly greater dose of thyroxine than those with hypothyroidism. A dose of 150 to 200 micrograms daily is usually enough to switch off TSH secretion by the pituitary gland.

HOW IS IT FOLLOWED UP?

Papillary and follicular cancers, like the normal thyroid gland, make a substance called thyroglobulin. The thyroid gland can secrete this substance only in the presence of TSH, but this is not the case with thyroid cancer. So, if there is no TSH detectable in the bloodstream because it has been suppressed by treatment with thyroxine, any thyroglobulin in the blood must be coming from recurrent cancer in the neck or from cancer that has spread to other parts of the body (secondaries or metastases). Thyroglobulin is therefore known as a 'tumour marker'. If a patient who is taking appropriate amounts of thyroxine has a raised level of thyroglobulin, the specialist may wish to perform a scan of the whole body using radioactive iodine to identify the site of the recurrent tumour or its metastases.

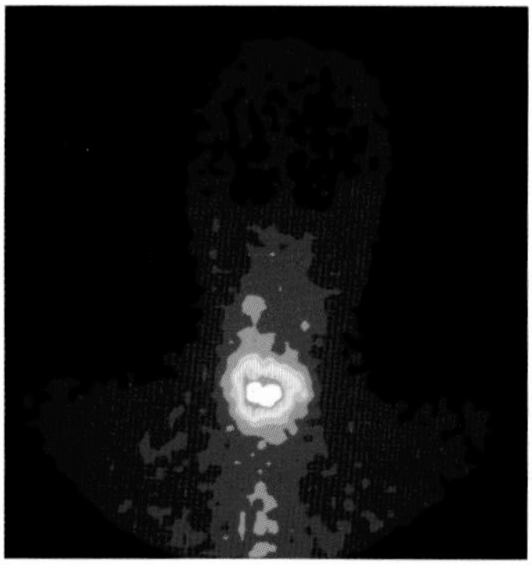

FINDING A TUMOUR
An isotope scan can identify the site of a recurrent tumour or its metastases. Cancerous cells are seen on this scan as white and yellow areas in the patient's neck.

The scan is usually performed 24 to 48 hours after a dose of iodine-131 by mouth, four weeks after the patient has stopped taking thyroxine or after TSH injections. Any tumour that is found may be treated with a large dose of radioactive iodine.

WHAT IS THE OUTLOOK?

The outlook depends upon the size of the tumour and whether it has spread at the time of diagnosis. If treated correctly, a young woman with a small papillary cancer of the thyroid is likely to have a normal life expectancy, despite the cancer having spread to the lymph nodes in the neck. Even patients with follicular cancer that has spread to the bones or lungs may survive for many years with a good quality of life.

Case History: **ENLARGED LYMPH NODES**

Susan Jones was 18 when she fell heavily, striking the side of her neck. As the pain and bruising settled she noticed a pea-sized lump in her neck. To begin with her doctor thought that it must be related to the accident, although it moved when she swallowed, suggesting that it lay within the thyroid gland.

When it hadn't disappeared after six weeks, he referred Susan to a thyroid specialist at the local teaching hospital. The consultant examined Susan's neck and found a single small thyroid nodule and three enlarged lymph nodes on the right side. He took a tiny sample from the thyroid nodule and from one of the lymph nodes, sucking out cells with a syringe and needle. The test took only a few minutes, causing Susan no discomfort and with no need even for a local anaesthetic.

The next day Susan was informed that the lump in her neck was a type of cancer of the thyroid, known as papillary carcinoma, and that it had spread to the nearby lymph nodes. Two weeks later Susan was admitted to hospital where almost all of her thyroid gland was removed, together with the enlarged lymph nodes. Careful inspection of the removed gland by the pathologists showed no other signs of thyroid cancer apart from the original swelling.

Susan has been cured and simply needs to take thyroxine tablets for the rest of her life and see the specialist every year for a blood test.

RARE CANCERS

Rarer forms of thyroid cancer include the following:

- Medullary cancer of the thyroid, which can occur on its own or may run in families in association with abnormalities of other endocrine glands or of the skeleton.
- Lymphoma of the thyroid, which usually affects elderly people and may be accompanied by evidence of disease in other parts of the body.
- Anaplastic cancer, which also affects elderly people.

The future prospects for people with these types of cancer is less good than for those with papillary or follicular cancer. Treatment is more difficult and may include chemotherapy and radiotherapy.

KEY POINTS

- Remember that thyroid cancer is rare.
- The two types of cancer that doctors most often see – papillary and follicular – can normally be treated successfully if they are caught early enough.
- Depending on the type, an operation is necessary to remove all or part of the thyroid gland, and those with papillary cancer may then need treatment with radioactive iodine to destroy any remaining cells.
- After surgery, patients will need to take thyroxine in slightly higher doses than normal.
- A blood test will probably be done after treatment to check that no trace of cancer remains and that it hasn't spread.
- There are a few very rare cancers that mainly affect elderly people, in whom treatment may be more difficult.

Thyroid blood tests

Increasingly, patients wish to know about the actual levels of thyroid hormones and thyroid stimulating hormone (TSH) in the blood. The normal or reference ranges for these hormones are shown in the box on p.62.

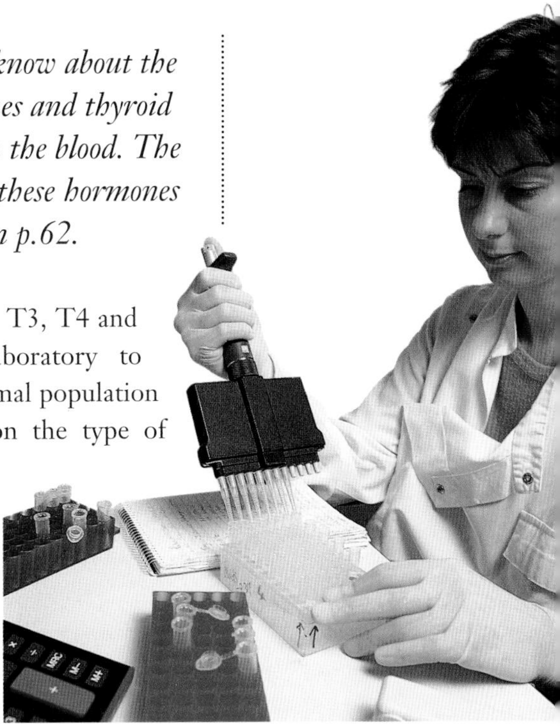

The normal or reference ranges for T3, T4 and TSH will vary slightly from laboratory to laboratory, depending upon the normal population used for the calculations, and upon the type of assay used for the measurement of the hormones. The thyroid hormones T3 and T4 are almost exclusively bound to a protein in the bloodstream and, as such, are inactive. Less than one per cent of these hormones is unbound or free and able to control the metabolism of the body.

LABORATORY TESTS
Tests are available to measure the levels of thyroid hormones and TSH in the blood.

Measurement of total T3 and T4 includes both bound and free fractions, whereas that of free T4 and T3 excludes the much larger bound fraction. Measurement of free and total thyroid hormones usually provides the same information on whether the thyroid is working normally or in an over- or underactive fashion. Some hospital laboratories offer measurement of total thyroid hormones and others offer free thyroid hormones, but rarely both.

Normal Hormone Reference Ranges

This table shows the normal reference ranges of thyroid hormones and TSH levels in the blood. Your GP or specialist will compare your blood tests with these figures to assess your condition.

HORMONE	REFERENCE RANGE
Total thyroxine (TT4)	60–150 nanomoles per litre (nmol/l)
Free thyroxine (fT4)	10–25 picomoles per litre (pmol/l)
Total triiodothyronine (TT3)	1.1–2.6 nanomoles per litre (nmol/l)
Free triiodothyronine (fT3)	3.0–8.0 picomoles per litre (pmol/l)
Thyrotrophin or thyroid-stimulating hormone (TSH)	0.15–3.5 milliunits per litre (mU/l)

nanomoles = 10^{-9} moles **picomoles = 10^{-12} moles**

For the scientifically minded, a mole is the molecular weight of a substance in grams.

- A mole of thyroxine is 777 grams.
- A nanomole of thyroxine is 777 nanograms (or 777×10^{-9} grams)
- A picomole of thyroxine is 777 picograms (or 777×10^{-12} grams).

Although most hormones are now measured in molar units, as this is thought to reflect activity more accurately, drugs are still prescribed in mass units or grams. A dose of 100 micrograms (or 100×10^{-6} grams) of thyroxine is the equivalent of about 130 nanomoles.

TYPICAL RESULTS

Generally speaking, the more severe the symptoms of over- or underactivity of the thyroid gland, the more abnormal the results of the thyroid blood tests. In most patients with hyperthyroidism, TT4 would be about 190 nmol/l, TT3 4.0 nmol/l, fT4 40 pmol/l and fT3 12 pmol/l. Much higher values may be recorded, however, with fT4 in excess of 100 pmol/l. In older patients, in whom hyperthyroidism may be no less serious, with heart complications such as an irregular heartbeat caused by atrial fibrillation, the levels of thyroid hormones may be only marginally elevated. In all patients with hyperthyroidism, with very rare exceptions, the TSH level in the blood is so low that it cannot be detected.

By the time that patients with hypothyroidism present with typical symptoms, fT4 and TT4 levels are very low and often less than 5 pmol/l and 20 nmol/l respectively, and associated with a raised TSH level in the blood of more than 30 mU/l. Rarely, hypothyroidism is the result of disease of the pituitary gland and not the thyroid gland itself, in which case the low fT4 or TT4 is combined with a normal or low level of TSH.

In mild or subclinical hypothyroidism (see p.36), fT4 and TT4 lie in the lower part of the normal range, e.g. 11 pmol/l or 65 nmol/l, and are usually associated with a TSH level in the blood of between 5 and 10 mU/l.

Levels of T3 are not usually measured in patients with suspected hypothyroidism.

JUDGING THE CORRECT DOSE

Your GP or thyroid specialist will usually prescribe a dose of thyroxine that raises the fT4 and TT4 to the upper part of the normal range and reduces the TSH level in the blood to the lower part of the normal range. Typical results would be fT4 of 24 pmol/l or TT4 of 140 nmol/l, and a TSH of 0.2 mU/l. In some patients, a sense of well-being is achieved only when fT4 or TT4 is raised, e.g. 30 pmol/l or 170 nmol/l, and TSH is low or undetectable. In this circumstance, it is essential that the T3 level in the blood is unequivocally normal in order to avoid hyperthyroidism.

If you are failing to take your thyroxine regularly, this will be very obvious from the blood test results.

EFFECT OF ILLNESS ON THYROID

Illness, whether sudden (such as pneumonia or a heart attack) or of long duration (such as rheumatoid arthritis or depression), may affect the results of thyroid blood tests and give the impression of hyper- or hypothyroidism. It is possible that, after referral to a specialist, and after further investigations, no underlying thyroid disease will be found.

Warning

Thyroid blood tests should not be interpreted in isolation, and correct medical care will also depend on careful assessment of symptoms and clinical examination.

KEY POINTS

- Different laboratories use slightly different normal ranges.
- The more severe the symptoms of thyroid malfunction, the more abnormal the blood test results will be.
- Blood test results enable the specialist to determine the necessary dose of thyroxine.
- Some other illnesses can produce thyroid blood test results that falsely suggest hyper- or hypothyroidism.

Questions and answers

Do I have to change my diet?

You may have heard that iodine has something to do with the thyroid gland. Indeed iodine is an integral part of the thyroxine (T4) and triiodothyronine (T3) molecules. A lack of iodine in the diet may cause a goitre or even hypothyroidism. This is commonly found in people who live in mountainous areas far from the sea, such as the Himalayas, but the diet in the UK contains adequate amounts of iodine and you don't need to take supplements. For the disbelievers, iodised salt is available in some supermarkets. Excessive iodine intake, however, may unmask underlying thyroid disease and produce either hyperthyroidism or hypothyroidism.

Is smoking harmful?

The eye disease that accompanies Graves' disease is more common and more severe among patients who smoke. Patients with hyperthyroidism caused by Graves' disease should stop smoking.

Was stress responsible for making my thyroid gland overactive?

Although it is difficult to prove, most thyroid specialists are impressed by how often major life events, such as divorce or death of a close relative, appear to have taken place a few months before the onset of hyperthyroidism caused by Graves' disease. There is now evidence that stress can affect the immune system, which is abnormal in Graves' disease. So the answer is probably 'yes', but there are other important factors, such as heredity.

Will my new baby have thyroid trouble?

The children of mothers with Graves' disease or a previous history of Graves' disease may be born with an overactive thyroid gland. This is known as neonatal thyrotoxicosis and lasts for only a few weeks. The obstetrician and the paediatrician will be looking out for this rare complication, which is readily treated. Occasionally, mothers with hypothyroidism give birth to a child with an underactive thyroid gland. Again this is usually short-lived and will be detected by the routine blood testing of all babies a few days after birth.

Will my children be affected?
Not necessarily. In fact, the risk is relatively small, although it is greater than that for children who have no family history of autoimmune disease. Nor is it always the same disease that runs in families. For example, a mother may have Graves' disease, while her daughter develops insulin-dependent diabetes mellitus.

Could my thyroid condition explain why I did badly in my exams?
It is likely to be hyperthyroidism that affects people who are the right age to be taking exams. If it is not adequately treated, a reduced ability to concentrate will certainly lead to a substandard performance and the specialist will be happy to write to the relevant headteacher or college tutor to explain the problem.

Could thyroid disease have caused my anxiety/depression?
The answer is almost certainly 'no', although hyperthyroidism and hypothyroidism will make underlying psychiatric illness worse. Unfortunately, even when a person who suffers from hyperthyroidism is successfully treated so that their overactive thyroid is brought under control, their psychiatric symptoms don't disappear altogether, although they may improve.

Will my Graves' disease recur?
If your hyperthyroidism has been effectively treated with iodine-131, it will never return. If the hyperthyroidism has settled after a single course of carbimazole there is a 30 to 50 per cent chance of recurrence, usually within one to two years of stopping the drug. Recurrent hyperthyroidism after surgery is usually apparent within a few weeks, but may occur as long as 40 years after apparently successful surgery.

Does it matter if I forget to take my medication?
The occasional missed tablet is not the end of the world. Indeed symptoms of hypothyroidism caused by lack of thyroxine are not usually felt for two to three weeks after stopping the tablets so it would still be possible to enjoy a seven to 10 day holiday if you'd inadvertently left your medication at home. However, this is not to be recommended. Also,

patients with hypothyroidism may have other autoimmune diseases such as diabetes mellitus. Failure to take thyroxine regularly will affect the response to insulin and may lead to unexpected coma as a result of low blood sugar.

Again, missing the odd carbimazole dose will not cause significant problems but symptoms of hyperthyroidism are likely to develop if you don't take the tablets for 24 to 48 hours, especially within a few weeks of starting treatment.

I feel better when I am taking a higher dose of thyroxine than recommended by my doctor. Is this safe?
There is considerable debate about the correct dose of thyroxine. The consensus is that enough should be given to ensure that levels of T4 in the blood are at the upper limit of normal or slightly elevated and TSH at the lower limit of normal, or in some patients undetectable. Although by taking excessive thyroxine, a sense of well-being, increased energy and even weight loss may be achieved in the short term, there are long-term dangers to the heart and a possibility of increasing the rate of bone thinning and therefore encouraging the development of osteoporosis.

Will tests involving radioactivity affect my fertility?
Definitely not. The amount of radioactivity involved is tiny – less than that in a X-ray so you have absolutely no cause for concern.

Can treatment for Graves' disease make me fat?
No, although you will probably put back any weight you lost before your condition was diagnosed and treated. However, there's no reason why you should end up weighing any more than you did before you started to develop Graves' disease.

My daughter was put on thyroxine tablets at birth because she was hypothyroid. Will she have to take them forever?
Not necessarily. She will be taken off them and then given a blood test when she's around one year old to see whether she still needs them.

Is the time of day when I take my thyroxine tablets important?
No, but most people find it's better to take them at the same time each day – that way you're less likely to forget. It does not matter when you take them in relation to meals.

Glossary

This glossary explains the meaning of the most frequently used clinical and related terms connected with the diagnosis and treatment of thyroid disorders.

antibodies: these are produced by the body's immune system as a defence mechanism against 'foreign' protein contained, for example, in bacteria. Antibodies are not normally formed against proteins that are part of the body.

autoimmune disease: inappropriate production of antibodies, which are directed against parts of the body. For example, in most patients with hypothyroidism, antibodies are formed that participate in the destruction of the thyroid gland. In Graves' disease, antibodies directed against the surface of the thyroid cell stimulate it to over-produce thyroid hormones.

carbimazole: the drug most commonly used in the UK in the treatment of hyperthyroidism. It acts by interfering with the excessive production of thyroid hormones.

de Quervain's thyroiditis: a form of viral thyroiditis that can occur following a viral infection of the thyroid.

exophthalmos: prominence of the eyes most commonly found in patients with hyperthyroidism caused by Graves' disease. The exophthalmos may affect one or both eyes, may be apparent before the overactive thyroid gland develops and may appear for the first time after successful treatment of the hyperthyroidism.

fine needle aspiration (FNA): a test that involves passing a small needle into the thyroid gland and sucking out (aspirating) a small sample of tissue for examination under the microscope. This technique often avoids the need for surgery in patients who have a certain type of goitre.

goitre: an enlarged thyroid gland.

Graves' disease: the name given to the most common form of hyperthyroidism. Patients often have exophthalmos, a goitre and sometimes raised red patches on the legs, known as pretibial myxoedema.

Hashimoto's thyroiditis: the name given to a particular kind of goitre caused by autoimmune disease. Although the thyroid gland is enlarged, there is often evidence of hypothyroidism.

hyperthyroidism: the condition resulting from an overactive thyroid gland.

hypothyroidism: the condition resulting from an underactive thyroid gland.

myxoedema: this means the same as hypothyroidism, but is often used to describe patients in whom the thyroid underactivity is severe and of long standing.

postpartum thyroiditis: a transient disturbance in the balance of the thyroid gland that can occur in the first year after childbirth. There are usually no symptoms, but there may be symptoms of hyperthyroidism or of hypothyroidism. Treatment is not usually necessary.

propranolol (Inderal): a drug belonging to the group known as beta-blockers, which alleviate some of the symptoms, e.g. tremor in patients with an overactive thyroid gland. Other members of the group include nadolol (Corgard) and sotalol (Sotacor).

proptosis: another word for exophthalmos.

propylthiouracil: this drug has a similar action to carbimazole. It is used if patients develop side effects to carbimazole and is prescribed to patients who are breast-feeding when hyperthyroid.

radioactive iodine (iodine-131): an isotope of iodine used in the investigation and treatment of hyperthyroidism.

tetany: this results from a low level of calcium in the blood with tingling in the hands, feet and around the mouth, and painful spasm of the muscles of the hands and feet.

thyroglobulin: a protein secreted by the thyroid gland. Its measurement is an important part of the follow-up of patients who have been treated for thyroid cancer. It is known as a 'tumour marker' because its presence in certain situations may indicate that the cancer has returned to other parts of the body.

triiodothyronine (T3): a hormone that, along with thyroxine, is secreted by the thyroid gland. It is responsible for controlling the metabolism of the body. Although available in tablet form, it is not usually prescribed for patients with hypothyroidism because it does not provide such good control as thyroxine.

thyrotoxicosis: another term for hyperthyroidism.

thyroxine (T4): a hormone secreted, along with triiodothyronine, by the thyroid gland. It has to be converted in the body to triiodothyronine before it is active. Thyroxine is available in tablet form for the treatment of hypothyroidism.

thyrotrophin (thyroid-stimulating hormone, TSH): a hormone, secreted by the pituitary gland, that is responsible for controlling the output of thyroid hormones by the thyroid gland. In hypothyroidism caused by disease of the thyroid gland, TSH concentrations are elevated in the blood and in hyperthyroidism TSH concentrations are low.

Useful addresses

British Thyroid Foundation
PO Box 97
Clifford,
Wetherby
West Yorkshire
LS23 6XD
The British Thyroid Foundation became a registered charity in 1991 and is run by volunteers who are committed to helping the thyroid disease sufferer. The principal aims of the Foundation are to provide support and clear information to sufferers of thyroid disorders, to promote a greater awareness of these disorders among the general public and the medical profession, to help to set up regional support groups and to raise funds for research.

Thyroid Eye Disease (TED)
34 Fore Street
Chudleigh
Devon
TQ13 0HX
Tel/fax: (01626) 852980

Index

Acknowledgements

PUBLISHER'S ACKNOWLEDGEMENTS

Dorling Kindersley would like to thank the following for their help and participation in this pr

Production Controller Michelle Thomas; **Con**
Indexing Indexing Specialists, Hove; **Administr**

Illustrations (p.8) ©Philip Wilson; (p

Picture Research Angela Anderson; **Picture I**

PICTURE CREDITS

The publisher would like to thank the following for their
photographs. Every effort has been made to trace the cop
apologises for any unintentional omissions and would
to add an acknowledgement in futu

National Medical Slide Bank p.10, p.56; **Science Pho**
p.26 (Dr. P.Marazzi), p.42 (Ron Sutherland),
p.58 (Oulette Theroux), p.61 (Sinclai